Table of Content

Copyright

Copyright© 2020 Jessica Robin

Author's Note and Disclaimer

The reader should consult their personal physician before beginning any weight loss program or changes in diet.

Discuss the information presented in this book with the Doctor / Physician / Professional trainer who knows you best before making any changes in diet / activity and before starting any weight loss plan

The content and information in this book has been taken from reliable sources, and it is accurate to the Author's knowledge. However, the Author is not a licensed practitioner or physician and the author cannot guarantee accuracy and validity of the content / information of the book.

The author claims no responsibility to any person or entity for any liability, loss or damage caused directly or indirectly as a result of the use, application, or interpretation of the content/information presented in this book.

The content and information in this book have been provided for educational purposes only.

Introduction

Welcome to the FAT OUT MAXIMUM WEIGHT LOSS! Over the past 50 years, obesity has increased, In one of the health survey for US and UK estimates that 40% of adults in the US and 29% of adults in England are obese and about 13-17% of the world's adult population are obese, and if we see the estimate about the men vs. women the survey estimates that 40% of women and 35% of men are obese in US, women are more likely suffering from obesity than men, and if we talk about children, 19% children ages between 2 to 18 are obese in US, and they are more likely to become obese adults, survey also estimates that the obesity costs $150 billion (20% of medical spending) each year in US, obesity is one of the primary reason for around 70 chronic diseases, and other health problems such as diabetes, heart disease, stroke and high blood pressure, that's way Obesity is considered a disease and like every disease we can control obesity too.

My goal in this book is to explain simple and safe way to lose unwanted pounds and shed ugly belly, hip, and thigh fat as quickly as possible without harmful side effects, extreme dieting, and teach you the different ways to get back in shape and stay that way, Inside this book you will find complete details about low-carb diet, body detoxification, Intermittent fasting, weight loss exercises at home and hundreds of healthy Home remedies, recipes, teas, smoothies etc. for overall good health and weight loss.

There are lot of benefits to losing weight, like, you will feel much healthier, more energetic, and look smarter and better than ever, even losing 5% of your body weight can have a good impact on your body.

Overweight! Why?

Lifestyle, eating habits, food quality and portion, age, general health and your genetic and physiological state also contribute to your weight.

Overeating

Your weight depends on the type of food you eat and the amount of food you eat, whether you exercise regularly and daily, whether the food is used to relieve stress, etc. We eat more calories than our bodies need in a day, so the excess calories are stored as fat.

many people tend to overeat, and it is a serious problem that causes a large number of people to become overweight or obese.

Consuming Quickly

If we eat faster, our brain does not know when to stop until it is too late. If we eat slowly, our brain has time to respond, which means we eat less because our stomach sends a message to our brain that I am full!

It also allows us to easily digest our food.

Lack Of Sleep

Most people generally sleep seven hours a night. But our weight will increase if we sleep less than eight hours a night. Why is it?

This is because the natural function of our body is threatened by lack of sleep. It can even stimulate the hormones that generate our appetite.

Genetic

It is a fact that you get your genetics from your parents and when they have a slow metabolism, which means that their bodies digest food very slowly than in most cases you may also have a slow metabolic rate.
But With focus and hard work, you can change this fact.

Metabolic Rate.

In addition to genetics, your metabolic rate depends on your activity. It is said that every ten years after the mid-twenties, we lose about 10% of our metabolism. However, this is probably not entirely related to age, but rather to our activity. The more active we are, the more muscle we can maintain or even develop, and the healthier we are because muscle tissue is metabolically active, but fat is not. Conversely, if we lead a sedentary life, we are much more likely to gain weight if we lose muscle.

Lack Of Activity And Movement

Activity and Exercise are important for a healthy lifestyle and to maintain a healthy weight. When you exercise, especially when you include strength training in your training, you gain muscle mass and increase your metabolism. The muscle helps burn more fat and appears thinner and firmer because muscles take up less space than fat. Strength training also helps reduce the risk of accidental injury, improve bone density, aid digestion, and lower blood pressure, cholesterol and triglycerides.

Health Risk Of Overweight

High blood pressure, blood lipids (triglycerides) and angina, which lead to serious heart problems and strokes. The problem occurs when plaque (a fatty material) builds up on the inner walls of the coronary arteries that supply the heart with oxygenated blood. The plaque in the arteries narrows them, reducing the flow of oxygenated blood to the heart.

As your BMI increases slowly, the chances of having heart attacks and diseases such as coronary artery disease increases.

In overweight people, the heart simply cannot pump enough blood into the circulatory system to meet the needs of the body, resulting in heart failure.

Strokes

if fat deposits in the arteries, which can lead to blood clots in the arteries. If the blocked artery is near the brain, it can block oxygen and blood flow to the brain, causing a stroke. Strokes are more common in people with a high BMI.

High Blood Pressure

This is due to the high pressure that the blood exerts when it presses against the walls of the arteries. Obese and overweight people are more likely to suffer from high blood pressure.

Arthritis

Arthritis is a problem in which the bone joint is stressed too much, It's not uncommon for older generations, but overweight young people will face this problem.

Depression

Depression is one of the most common mental health problems in overweight people. Because of their size, they are usually the primary target of bullying, jokes and criticism. It also leads to lower self-esteem.

Cancer

In the United States, the second deadliest disease that kills thousands of people is cancer. Many types of cancer may develop if you are overweight or obese.

Cancer is common in men as colon, rectum and prostate cancer, while cancer of the breast, colon, ovaries, gallbladder, uterus and cervix uteri are common in women.

Gallbladder Stones

Obese people may have problems such as inflamed gallbladder and small stones in the gallbladder. These small stones, which are usually caused by high cholesterol, cause abdominal pain and the only remedy available is surgery.

Diabetes

Non-insulin diabetes mellitus (also called type II diabetes) is common in the United States. This affects the body by reducing its ability to control the level of blood sugar. Obese people are twice as likely to develop diabetes as people with average weight. Diabetes cannot be cured completely, so people who suffer from it must take a daily dose of the medication. This disease can also lead to complications and other health problems such as blindness, heart problems, strokes and kidney failure.

Sleep Apnea

This is another problem related to obesity. People with sleep apnea stop breathing for a short period of sleep. This often leads to drowsiness day and night

Liver Damage

If there is too much fat in the liver, the liver may suffer from scarring, inflammation, or even permanent liver damage.

Polycystic Ovary Syndrome

Obese women can suffer from polycystic ovary syndrome, in which they miss their period or have no period at all. This can lead to an excess of testosterone hormones that cause acne, excessive hair growth and even baldness. The testosterone hormone also disrupts ovulation and causes infertility.

When you look at all of the health complications associated with overeating and a sedentary lifestyle, you shouldn't be surprised that most overweight people are as young as 60. When they realize it, the need for a diet becomes obvious and they want to do something before it is too late for them.

Basics Of Weight Loss

If you are overweight, the weight loss should be gradual and regular. The process should not be speeded up and you should never lose more than 10 pounds per week. It is the safest way to lose weight.

If you want to lose weight effectively, you won't find a magic pill or drink to lose weight without seriously changing your lifestyle and diet

It's sad but true! Marketers know that everyone wants to lose weight and feel good without a lot of work.

Always ignore products that promise results for which you don't have to make an effort. Losing weight requires diet, work, exercise and a health program, without these activities it is quite difficult.

How Diets Work?

Losing weight is easy; lose more calories than you eat.

We eat because it is necessary. The food we eat is processed by our body, breaks it down and keeps only what we need while the rest is thrown away. While we perform our normal daily tasks, our body uses the calories and nutrients from our food to fuel our body to perform all day long. However, our body only needs a certain amount of calories, which means that all the unused calories are stored as fat in our body.

The problem with our body is that there is no way to tell it to stop storing calories. All the excess calories are converted to fat, no matter how much fat you already have in your body. Most of us always eat more than we need and ingest all those extra calories to become overweight.

Basically diet is supposed to help you lose those extra calories.

A diet is a nutritional plan in which you control the amount of calories consumed. Eating less is not the only way to diet. Since the goal is to eat fewer calories, you can eat consistently, but it is low in calories. Foods like fruits or vegetables are low in calories.

If you are on a diet, you are eating less than normal. It will make you hungry all day and you will feel more dissatisfied after you finish your meal. It cannot be avoided because you are at least trying to reduce your calorie intake. But in this book you will find some delicious and low in calories recipes, you will not feel hungry anymore.

This is to make sure that you can adhere to the diet plan for the duration and reach your goal. Diet plans also give you alternative snacks that you can eat to suppress your cravings.

This book also included low calorie snacks, soup, salad, smoothie, tea and much more.

If you're on a diet, don't think you'll have water and vegetables all day. The diet actually promotes eating a balanced meal. You just want to have fewer calories, but the rest of the nutrients should not be overlooked.

So if you avoid certain types of food, you also avoid their nutrients. The diet therefore shows you alternative foods that you can take to replace the missing nutrients. These foods are generally avoided and are not completely banned. So you can still eat them in small portions from time to time.

Metabolism

Good nutrition also contributes to your natural metabolism. Everyone has their own metabolic rate. A person with a higher metabolic rate can burn more calories per day. A proper diet can help people with low metabolism take full advantage of it.

Like a real breakfast to boost your metabolism, a lunch to keep your energy running and less to eat at dinner because you don't burn as many calories at night. This is to make sure that you have enough calories for the day.

Calorie Calculator

how many calories you burn naturally each day. It depends on factors such as age and weight.

Calculate the number of calories you burn each day

BMR Men (weight in pounds)
BMR = 66 + (6.23 x weight) + (12.7 x height in inches) – (6.76 x age in years)

BMR Women (weight in pounds)
BMR = 655 + (4.35 x weight) + (4.7 x height in inches) – (4.7 x age in years)

This formula gives you the basic calories you burn daily just by breathing, heart pumps, etc. These are the calories you burn when you haven't moved all day.

Once you have that number, you need to start tracking the calories burned.

This can be difficult because a lot of information must be kept in mind.

There are websites where you can track. Just enter the foods and activities you had for the day. You can even enter your basal metabolic rate BMR.

This is ideal if you can maintain a daily calorie deficit, but it is not always possible. Sometimes we slip and sometimes we spoil ourselves with something. If you have a weekly calorie deficit, you will still lose weight.

It's not about starving yourself or exercising until you die. It's about being aware of what you put in your body.

Negative Calories

Losing weight is always tied to eating less. It is because you need to have negative calories by the end of the day. It is counted by having the total calories that you eat in a day minus the amount of calories you burn. While the amount of calories burnt per person varies, the general idea is a person would burn 2000 calories a day just surviving. This means the organ is working, functioning brain and you are breathing.

So to have lower than 2000 calories a day, you need to limit your food intake. This is so you would take fewer calories per day. You might think that only by limiting your food intake that is the only way to achieve that. That idea works but it is already considered outdated. There is a new diet plan that lets you eat all that you want, keeping your stomach full but still keep the calories count in check. This is really eating yourself to a slimmer figure.

Clean Food

We talked about calories, the basic guideline for weight loss. This is basic advice because you always want to make sure you get those calories from good sources. Keeping your calories low by eating two corn dogs a day is probably not your best bet.

Eating clean is a term, in general it means:"Eat healthy whole foods, avoiding processed foods and refined sugar."This is a general objective which must be sought. It is not always possible to eat completely clean. However, if you get most of your calories from clean sources, it's fine. When you eat healthy, you avoid processed foods then foods like fast food and junk food are automatically removed from your diet. If you eat processed food, don't worry. The idea is to eat as lean as possible.

Here are some general tips for clean food:

- Learn to read labels! Read the nutritional information and ingredients of everything you buy.
- If possible, choose whole grain products
- Eat lots of fruits and vegetables. They are great sources of clean calories
- Prepare more of your own meals.
- Choose lean meat when cooking. Eating meat is good and protein helps build muscle and makes you feel full. Chicken and fish are a good selection of meats.
- Avoid processed meats like Bologna or hot dogs.
- Replace junk food with whole unsalted or lightly salted nuts.

Eating clean is a great way to make sure you're not only losing weight, but eating for overall health. It is not easy to choose clean food but if you want to lose weight and be healthy, you should choose a clean diet.

Portion Control

Anyone trying to lose weight should control the portion. Just talk to anyone who has actually lost weight. You will almost certainly approach portion control as one of the keys to success.

What is portion control?

Portion control means understanding how much a serving is and how many calories a serving contains.

When you eat a meal, check your portions! Learning the amount of food you really need, is one of the biggest steps you will take to lose weight.

Distributing meals in smaller portions instead of eating huge meals is an important factor in losing weight. It has been proven that rationing your meals not only reduces your calorie intake throughout the day, but also helps stabilize your metabolism. If you are used to eating 2 or 3 massive meals a day, you should eat 6 to 7 small meals spread throughout the day.

One thing people like to do is eat straight out of the package instead of taking what they need and putting away the package. One such example is to eat from a packet of large potato chips. Not only do you have idea how much you are consuming, but you usually respond to a craving by eating more than you really need until you are completely satisfied. Super-big packages are more common today, More items are sold in bulk and more groceries are served in restaurants with the option of increasing the size for a few extra cents. Increased proportions are a factor in the increase in obesity statistics. There is always a reason, but people put pleasure above everything else, which of course carries a health risk.

It takes discipline to make adjustments, and there is really no reason for people to feel like they are eating until they are full. As always, tiny portions are fine, and if they're still spicy, add a little more instead of loading your plate and trying to finish it off.

This helps control the weight and slowly begins to drop. It is a wonderful feeling when you experience it. This motivates you to work a little harder because you are sure that you can take control of your own body rather than letting your desire take control of you.

Water

Research has shown that you need at least 8 glasses of water a day. However, it can depend on your weight, how much you actually need. You should cut your weight in half so that, for example, a 180 pound man needs 60 ounces of water a day.

Why do experts suggest drinking lots of water and why is it considered so important for healthy living?

First of all, it helps prevent dehydration and the kidneys work well by helping to eliminate waste. It also helps increase metabolism and lose weight. But other than what the experts tell you, listening to your body first should be a priority. Of course, if you are thirsty, drink water to replenish it.

Depending on the type of work you do, try to get used to drinking water regularly or better: A bottle of water, especially in very hot weather, as you sweat through the heat and your body loses water and you need to recharge.

This is why water is so important in our lives. Not only is it calorie-free, it is also the best source to quench your thirst. You can consider adding water to all your meals over time and ultimately leaving fruit drinks and sodas aside as this will help you reduce your calorie intake and make you feel much better without the added sugar that accompanies other drinks.

make sure to not drink water just before food or just after, keep the gap of minimum 20 minutes between food and water, 40 minutes gap is recommended.

Junk Food

Cut all the junk food

The next thing you need to do is to cut all the garbage. We have seen that it is only empty calories that make us hungry - so stop eating them!

and make sure to limit the consumption of carbohydrates such as white bread, white pasta or bars of chocolate. You can also do this by largely following a natural carbohydrate diet.

Low-carb Diet
What is low-carb diet?

We often hear about low-carb diets and their effectiveness in losing weight, but what is a low-carb diet?

The term "low carbohydrate" means low carbohydrate. Carbohydrates are usually found in foods such as pasta, potatoes, fruit, bread and rice. A low-carb diet does not include a specific diet or clearly defined steps to lose weight.

It is a rather vague term, which varies according to the person who uses it. However, some common characteristics are the consumption of foods low in carbohydrates and low blood sugar. The body excretes insulin through the consumption of carbohydrates.

When carbohydrates are digested, glucose - the effect of insulin secretion - is burned by our body when we need energy immediately, or it is stored as fat.

Seriously, after a meal consisting mainly of carbohydrates, the level of insulin in our body suddenly increases and suddenly decreases after a short time. This effect means that we are not hungry until 2 or 4 hours after our last meal, which leads to a vicious cycle in which we are hungry, then eat and finally store the fat.

The main way to define a low-carb diet is to answer the first question: "What is a low-carb diet?" Indicate whether you are talking about the actual carbohydrates an adult consumes daily or the percentage of a person's dietary calories derived from carbohydrates.

The usual amount of calories allowed in the diet of an adult is about 50 to 60%. Any percentage of calories from carbohydrates below that can be considered low in carbohydrates.

The most common misconception about low-carb diets is that people who follow this type of diet actually try not to eat carbs. Not only is this wrong, but it is also almost impossible because carbohydrates are hidden in most of the foods we eat, especially processed foods.

A low-carbohydrate diet, as the name suggests, tries to reduce carbohydrates to a low level and not eliminate them completely.

Another common myth is that a low-carb diet prohibits you from eating fruits and vegetables. The truth is that this food category is high in carbohydrates, but that doesn't mean you have to eliminate it.

It comes from his diet. Fruits and vegetables are the carbohydrates that should be eaten with a diet that contains little but no carbohydrates.

The main benefits of low-carbohydrate diets are weight loss and increased energy. People are less sleepy and have better concentration. Some cases have shown people to be in a better mood.

Bad thoughts and feelings seem to be seriously reduced or eliminated. You cannot overstate the positive results of low carb eating habits. People have noticed improvements in their metabolism, an advantage that is seen as a boost to a diet that focuses on weight loss, even if the weight loss is initially insignificant. A change in metabolism is essential on the path to a healthy path

The Benefits Of Low-carb Diet

When choosing a diet, you want to make sure that there are many positive benefits in addition to losing weight. Overall, you want to be healthier by eating, because the diet dictates that you eat every day. You also want to be able to follow the life plan instead of a few weeks or months. The benefits of a low-carb diet are offered by the healthy daily program, which you can implement for life. You will not see that eating carbohydrates will increase health problems. By reducing the daily volume of carbohydrates you eat, some common illnesses may be cured. like the frequency of headaches, joint pain, and difficulty concentrating decreases as you eat less carbohydrates. This can help reduce the amount of pain reliever you take when the headache and joint pain subsides. You'll feel healthier and save money on drugs with the benefits of a low-carb diet.

If you're on a diet, mood swings can often occur. The ups and downs of mood and energy can lead to binge eating. Another benefit of a low-carb diet is the balance between mood and energy. In fact, the body gets more energy from proteins and other nutrients than carbohydrates. Carbohydrates cause short-term energy explosions that quickly lower your energy level once the carbohydrates are digested. By reducing the volume of carbohydrates you eat, your energy is derived from other nutrients that contain more uniform energy that reduces mood and energy fluctuations.

If you like to exercise and want to strengthen and build muscles to fight the fat in your body, a low-carb diet can help.

After workout, your muscles are very sensitive to insulin and don't need as many carbohydrates as some people might think. With a low-carbohydrate diet, your muscles absorb more amino acids from your meal after workout. Amino acids help muscles heal faster from exercise and burn more fat.

The effects or prevention of diabetes can be supported by a low-carbohydrate diet. If you have diabetes, a low-carb diet can help you better balance your insulin levels throughout the day. If you have family members with diabetes and want to prevent the onset of the disease, a low-carb diet is a good, healthy way to naturally balance your insulin.

As you can see, a low-carbohydrate diet offers many benefits beyond weight loss. You will notice an improvement in your weight loss plan, but you will also have more energy and you will feel healthier. It is also the goal of losing weight; to be healthier.

Eating more vegetables and protein as well as fruits and nuts can be a good start for a low-carb diet. Gradually reduce your intake of bread, candy and items made from white flour and white sugar. You can find many free recipes for low carb diets on blogs, websites and TV shows for food preparation.

Are Low-carb Diets Safe?

Obesity is the most common problem in the world, it has attracted so much attention in recent times that the concept of weight loss has opened thousands of lucrative business opportunities. This marketing seems to have a negative impact on actual weight loss.

Calorie intake and calorie burning, the two main variables in the weight loss equation, A low carbohydrate diet has proven to be the solution for maintaining variable calorie intake in certain amounts. How it helps you lose weight is simple logic. As soon as the intake decreases, the body begins to use the stored fat, which results in weight loss. Sure, it will cause weight loss, but will it be a safe process?

The answer is not a simple yes or no. Although weight loss experts continue to emphasize the importance, nutritionists and the medical community disagree. It is widely believed that no matter how effective the results, side effects will disrupt body functions if carbohydrates are not cut in moderate amounts. Not only moderate, but also the right choice.

For example, reducing your fat intake without paying attention to the type of fat can even lead to an increase in blood cholesterol. You must have sufficient knowledge to determine what should and should not be included. Here, according to the example, a well-designed diet would have included polyunsaturated fats and monounsaturated fats, which are considered safe.

The same theory applies to all nutrients as to fat. Some diets even recommend avoiding fruits and vegetables. Such plans are harmful. Limiting fruits like bananas or watermelons with high blood sugar levels could at least make sense to support this plan. However, limiting all types of fruits and vegetables is baseless advice that worsens your health.

Reduced consumption of calcium-rich foods such as whole grains can even cause serious illnesses such as osteoporosis. Women with calcium deficiencies tend to have menstrual cramps. Most low-carb diets focus more on protein intake. Unnecessary amounts of protein force the kidneys to work harder to remove excess protein waste. The accumulation of harmful waste can cause kidney stones.

The most important thing is to understand your body well before choosing a diet. A kidney patient should pay attention to protein, while a heart patient should focus more on fat. There are also many factors to consider before following a low-carb diet.

Changes in your lifestyle also require changes in your eating plans. When you start exercising or building weights, your body's energy needs are different from what they were. Or if you have become pregnant, the changes should take place immediately. In such cases, advice is essential.

Extremely low-carbohydrate diets may not be safe. But take them on a "real carbohydrate" diet and get the slim body you've always dreamed of being healthy.

Common Mistakes About Low-carb Diet

Some people assume that a low-carbohydrate diet simply means eating meat every day. It is wrong; Everyone needs to know how to cut down on carbohydrates, what is high-carbohydrate foods, and what is a low-carb diet?.

Lack of sufficient fat This could be mistaken for a low-carbohydrate diet because you think low-carb is low-fat. People can start a low-fat diet, but over time it will consume their own body fat and starve very quickly. Therefore, it is important that you add fat to your body during a low-carbohydrate diet.

Lack of sufficient vegetables - With a low-carbohydrate diet, some people often forget to include vegetables and fruits in their diet. This will ultimately be catastrophic, since vegetables and fruits must be eaten in large quantities in a low-carbohydrate diet, especially fruits with low sugar content.

Eat too much - There is no point in counting the amount of calories in a low-carb diet. This does not mean that you should keep eating and eating just because he or she is eating low carb foods. It is recommended to eat only when you are hungry and to stop when you are satisfied.

Poor planning - Sometimes sticking to a new nutrition program can be a problem, and you may find that it does what it did before. It is therefore recommended to plan in advance to facilitate the free adoption of new eating habits. It means you know what and when to eat what.

Packaged Foods

Using low-carb packaged foods

When purchasing low-carb packaged foods, it is very important to understand the ingredients. Most of them contain maltitol, a bad sugar. Therefore, these low-carbohydrate foods should be carefully tested.

Lack of variety - Most people find a limited selection of low-carb foods, but there are many. The only thing you should avoid with a low carb diet is sugar and starch. Every kitchen on the planet has a low-carb selection; Most dishes can also be decarburized.

Insufficient fiber - If you eat vegetables and fruit, you can eat enough fiber. However, forgetting or missing vegetables and fruit reduces the amount of fiber in the body and can be catastrophic in the long run.

Carbs Against Fats

At this point, you may be wondering why carbohydrates are the main source of glucose in your diet when fats actually contain many more calories ...

The answer is that it depends on how the body uses these calories. And this is one of the causes of complications and arguments in the fitness industry.

You see, the body can gain energy from carbohydrates much faster than any other food. This is especially true for "simple carbohydrates" like candy and white bread (complex carbohydrates - including rye bread and sweet potato - work more like fat).

So if you eat a large plate of carbohydrates, your blood sugar will rise immediately. This in turn leads to the sudden release of large amounts of insulin, which forces the body to absorb glucose from the blood and ultimately store it as fat.

This in turn leads to hypoglycemia (and consequently low serotonin level), which makes you feel tired, and hungry. Fats, on the other hand, release their 9 grams of sugar into the bloodstream much more slowly and provide them with a more uniform and sustainable energy supply without the crash. Fats are also present in the stomach and ensure that you feel full for longer.

They can actually slow down the digestion of simple carbohydrates when eaten at the same time, and they can improve the absorption of nutrients. In fact, many supplements require that you eat them with a source of saturated fat to facilitate absorption.

For example, if you eat lutein to improve your eyesight and energy efficiency, you should take it with whole milk!

foods that reduce fat can also significantly reduce their calorie content. For example, a diet tuna sandwich contains 50 to 100 calories less than a store-bought sandwich. So you can lose weight.

At the same time, removing fat from food means that energy hits faster and harder and that you absorb fewer nutrients. It still makes you hungry. It can also mean that you get less food to build a strong, healthy body and mind.

And that's before you even think about the health benefits that fat directly has. For example, fat is an important building block of the brain and is used by the body to produce testosterone which increases metabolism and helps build muscle.

Good Carbohydrate

Natural carbohydrate is in most foods that is natural like oatmeal, potatoes and whole wheat. The foods are still in their natural state and have not been processed or refined severely by machines or people. Foods containing natural carbohydrates also contain a lot of fiber which gives you a lot of energy over a long period of time. This in turn keeps you feeling full for a longer period. High fiber foods also help in lowering cholesterol. Natural carbohydrates are also classified as low in the Glycemic index. So the glucose released by natural carbohydrates are lower and this fact is important to diabetics.

Bad Carbohydrate

Bad carbohydrates can be found in foods that are already refined. Most of the time, the most of the nutritional value is removed and they are loaded with colorings, preservatives and flavorings. They are popular with people because they come in nice packaging and are full of flavors. In turn they are hard to digest and cause a spike of glucose when it is digested. You do not benefit much from eating that food because they only provide mostly bad carbohydrates. One may feel energetic after eating them but it is only temporary. To continue feeling energetic, one would want to eat more and lead to more calories in take.

Good Fat

Like carbohydrates, fats also exist in its good form and bad form. Good fats are monounsaturated fat and polyunsaturated fat. Monounsaturated fat has lower total cholesterol and LDL cholesterol who clogs accumulates and clogs your arteries while are high in HDL cholesterol who carries cholesterol from the artery walls and into your liver to be disposed of. Most nuts and olive oil contain a lot of monounsaturated fat.

Polyunsaturated fat also has lower total cholesterol and LDL cholesterol. The beneficial Omega -3 fatty acids belong to this category. We cannot produce this Omega-3 so we have to eat them to have it. Foods like salmon, canola oil and linseed contain a lot of polyunsaturated fat.

Bad Fat

Bad fat is divided into two categories, saturated fat and trans fat. Saturated fat is mostly found in animal products like meat, eggs, dairy, and seafood. These fats are solid at room temperature. They have a lot of total cholesterol and LDL cholesterol.

The worst fat of all is trans fat. Trans fats are fat that went through a hydrogenation process where liquid vegetable oil is converted into solid fat. They are made so manufacturers can make food that has longer shelf life. Not only do they have the most total cholesterol and LDL cholesterol, trans fat also lowers HDL cholesterol. So processed food like margarine contains a lot of trans fat.

Now that you have a better understanding of both carbohydrate and fat, you can begin to see how you can eat yourself to this. All you need to do is to take note of what food you're currently eating has bad carbohydrates and fat so you can replace them with food that is high with good carbohydrates and fat. I will guide you through this so you can get a better understanding of the food to avoid or eat less while eating more beneficial food without worries.

Another problem that you would face when trying to replace your daily meal is that you do not know how to cook them. Anyone can learn how to make salad or bread but to make them healthy and low on calories is another problem. I have already included a few recipes that you can read to get a head start in your diet. Do not be restricted to general food sources for your diet. Even though it is recommended to eat a lot of vegetables and fruits, this does not mean you have to eat salad for a year. You can do a variety of dishes like stir-fry, soups or make desserts with them. Have a variety in your diet; it will keep you from feeling sick from eating all the vegetables and fruits.

Below is a general list of food that contains bad carbohydrate:
- White Pasta
- White Rice
- White Bread
- Instant Oatmeal
- Fruit Juices
- Bagels
- Donuts
- Muffins
- Sweets and Candies
- Processed Breakfast Cereals

These are the foods that you should avoid or not eat regularly. One of the simplest ways to know what food contains bad carbohydrates is to know if the food is processed or not. If it is, then usually it contains a lot of bad carbohydrates.

Good food that you can eat regularly is:
- Any fruits or vegetables
- Oatmeal
- Brown rice
- Potatoes
- Wheat products
- Wholegrain cereals
- High fiber breakfast cereals
- Grits
- Muesli
- Cassava
- Corn
- Amaranth
- Navy beans
- Whole Barley
- Buckwheat / Buckwheat pasta

So if you replace your daily bad carbohydrate with good carbohydrate, then you can eat more while not gaining more weight. Also you would feel full for much longer, suppressing your need to eat. Diet plans usually already include low carbohydrate recipes so you would gain even less daily if you replace them all in the good carbohydrate list.

Nutrient-rich Foods

Look for nutrient-rich foods

look for foods that provide a source of strong and useful nutrients.

A good example of this is something like organ meat which is filled with incredible nutrients. You get not only all the amino acids from meat, but also high amounts of creatine, CoQ10, PQQ and fatty acids. It makes sense if you think about it again: these are the most important and complex parts of these animals, and they again consist of things similar to the most complex and important parts of your own body.

Likewise, eating eggs, fish, tropical fruits and vegetables, and sea plants helps provide your body with all kinds of important nutrients. Be sure to mix it all with carbohydrates or complex fiber to slow the absorption of nutrients, and be sure to add low calorie oil or consume another source of saturated fat to aid absorption.

This is another reason why the Mediterranean diet looks good on paper - because it contains a lot of salads, a lot of superfoods, a lot of fish and everything that is filled with lots of nutrients.

If you strive to do this, you will now have a much better diet and will be energized and protected from disease. At the same time, you will really enjoy your meals and you will not feel hungry or cravings!

Good Nutrient, Bad Nutrient

Foods that we take are digested. Beneficial nutrients will be absorbed; the rest will be taken out. Even in those nutrients, there are some that you would want to have less of it when you are dieting. Carbohydrates and fats are the two main nutrients that you would want to avoid.

Carbohydrate is one of the main sources of energy. It will be broken down into glucose and be absorbed by the cells as food. If you introduce too much carbohydrate one time into your body, then you will get an insulin spike and a prolonged effect will cause diabetes.

Fat despite the general view of society plays an important factor in our body. Not only is it one of the main sources of energy, it also helps in absorbing Vitamins A, D, E, and K. Without them, you can't receive those vitamins at all. So if you are a growing teenager, it is not advisable that you completely skip food that contains fat unless it is specified by your doctor.

Since our body requires carbohydrates and fats but the diets want to limit our intake of those two, I bet you are wondering how you are going to eat yourself too thin. The answer simply lies in your choice of food. Even in those carbohydrates and fats, there are the good kinds and the bad kinds. So naturally we would want to control our intake of the good nutrients and avoid the bad.

Weight Loss with Herbs, Vitamins And Minerals

Some herbs are also known to have beneficial effects on certain bodily functions such as digestion, metabolism, Boost immunity, improve heart health, control blood sugar or to help curb the appetite to impact weight loss. There are a wide variety of herbs and herbal compounds that can boost your efforts to lose weight. Let's consider a few herbs that can help supplement your weight loss efforts:

Garcinia Cambogia

Promotes Weight Loss, Improves Metabolism, Increases Energy, Suppresses Appetite, Reduces Stress, Helps with Depression, Lowers Cholesterol, Regulates Blood Sugar

Cinnamon

Diabetes Management, Anticancer Potential, Boost Mental Health, Boost Bone Health, Increase cognitive ability, Improve heart health, Improve Digestive Health, Prevent bacterial infections, Treat common cold and flu

Nutmeg

Relieves Pain, Relieves Insomnia, Promotes Digestion, Improves Brain Health, Boost Oral Health, Protect Liver, Regulates Blood Pressure, Anticancer Potential, Boost health of the skin, Lowers LDL Cholesterol Levels, Giving relief from diarrhea, Prevent spread of seizures,

Ginger

Treats Cold and Flu, Relieves Nausea, Aids in Digestion, Removes Excess Gas, prevents Stomach Ulcers, Reduces

Arthritis Pain, Relieves Asthma, Prevent hepatotoxicity, Aid in the prevention of cancer, Improves Cognition, Relieves Muscle Pain, Reduce weight, Prevents Menstrual Cramps, Boosts Heart Health, Controls Diabetes, Detoxifies the Body, Prevents Infection, Treats Diarrhea, Increases Sexual Activity,

Cloves

Improve digestion, Reducing flatulence, gastric irritability, Control lung cancer, Control blood sugar levels, Helpful in preserving bone density, Immunity Booster, Reduce pain and inflammation, Care gum diseases,

Lemon

Manages Hypertension, Aids Weight Loss, Prevents Kidney Stones, Care gum infection, Care Hair loss, damage, dandruff, Cure sunburns, acne, eczema, Make skin glowing and lighten, Soothes Respiratory Disorders, Fights throat infections,

Black Pepper

prevent tumor, Cure breast, colorectal, prostate cancer, Improves Digestion, Reduce weight, Provide relief from vitiligo, Provides Respiratory Relief, Helps fight against infections, insect bites, Enhances Bioavailability, Improves Cognition, Gives Relief from Peptic Ulcers, Prevents Asthma, Control weight,

Cumin Seeds

Boosts Immunity, Improves Memory, Increases Lactation, Soothes Inflammation, Fights Common Cold, Prevent cancer, Lowers Cholesterol, Reduces the Risk of

Diabetes, Relieves Respiratory Disorders, Rich in Iron, Regulates Digestion.

Trachyspermum Ammi

Reduces Weight, Aid in Digestion, Reduce Acidity, Boost Respiratory Health, Relieve Asthma, Strengthen Immune System, Prevent Chronic Diseases, Give Relief from Headache, Prevent a Toothache, Prevent Formation of Kidney Stones, Reducing Pain of Piles, And Regulates Blood Pressure

Cayenne

Yes, this is the same tongue burning chili. Cayenne contains capsaicin, which has proved to stimulate digestion and increase metabolism, as well fat burning.

Seaweed

Seaweed or kelp stimulates metabolism. It is also a natural thyroid stimulant – which in turn is great help in losing weight.

Ginseng

Ginseng is known to stimulate your rate of metabolism and boost energy at the same time

Hoodia Gordonii

The herb hoodia gordonii has recently gained much attention as a weight loss aid. It is commonly called hoodia. The hoodia plant is grown in the desert regions of Africa and has been used by the peoples of the Kalahari for centuries.

Hoodia's Modus Operandi

Hoodia's modus operandi is to suppress your appetite, and research by Brown University in the USA has shown that hoodia interrupts or stops the hunger mechanism in the brain.

Green Tea

We have mentioned green tea as a supplement that helps weight loss, but let's look at it a little bit more closely.

Studies show that the caffeine and polyphenols in green tea speed up the rate at which calories are burned, and hence raise the metabolism.

Raising metabolism causes the body to burn more calories which of course leads to weight loss. Research has also indicated that green tea consumption creates a higher rate of fat oxidation, which can also help weight loss. Other benefits of green tea are Delay signs of aging, improve blood circulation, Increases Energy, Powerful Stimulating Effect, Boosts Immunity, Toning up muscles and skin, Anticancer Potential, Improves Cardiac & Arterial Health, Controls Diabetes , Boosts Stamina & Endurance, Detoxifies the Body.

Lutein

Lutein A lesser known carotenoid that is found in the macula of the eye. This is a great micronutrient for reducing the likelihood of impaired vision as you reach older age and can also do a lot of other things. Lutein is linked with energy efficiency and in studies it has been shown to help rats lose weight and run further on their volition.

Choline

Choline is a crucial nutrient found in eggs. This is the precursor to a chemical used in the brain known as 'acetylcholine'. Acetylcholine is the brain's principle neurotransmitter used for communication between cells. The more acetylcholine you have in your brain, the more focused, alert and awake you are. Supplementing has been shown to boost memory, IQ and more!

Creatine

Creatine is a wonder-substance that is incredibly useful for a wide range of different purposes and which is popularly used among athletes. The main role of creatine is to help the cells recycle used ATP to provide you with a few seconds of extra energy. This allows you to run faster for longer and to live heavier items. Once again, it has also been shown to improve attention and concentration!

Omega 3 Fatty Acid

Omega 3 fatty acid is an antioxidant that can help to protect cells from damage by free radicals and oxidants. This means that it can help to fight the effects of ageing, while at the same time reducing the likelihood of cancer. At the same time, omega 3 fatty acid can also improve the communication between cells by improving 'cell membrane permeability'. This can help to improve IQ. Omega 3 is also great for healthy skin and joints.

Casein

Casein is a great type of protein found in milk. Unlike whey, casein releases slowly which makes it ideal to consume before bed. This way, you will be given a steady and constant supply of protein as you are in your most 'anabolic' state during sleep

Tryptophan

Found in numerous proteins and other foods, tryptophan is a natural precursor to serotonin – what we know as the 'happiness hormone'. This can fight depression, boost your mood and even help you to sleep better at night.

Shilajit

This is an awesome example of the kind of 'powerup' you can get from the wild if you know where to look and how to hunt it down. Shilajit is a nutrient-rich that can be found oozing from between rocks high in mountain crevasses throughout India. This stuff has been shown to boost cellular energy and provide antioxidant and energy benefits. In India it is often referred to as 'the destroyer of weakness'.

Zinc

Zinc is implicated in neuroplasticity. That means that it makes it easier to learn new skills and abilities. What's more is that it also helps to increase testosterone production and improves function of the central nervous system. Many people have a deficiency in zinc.

Acetyl-l-carnitine

This is an amino acid that increases mitochondrial function and thereby enhances brain energy metabolism. It is often given to people suffering with chronic fatigue syndrome. That's right – each of the 20 amino acids that we need also provides other crucial functions in the body!

Nitric Oxide

Nitric oxide helps to improve blood flow around the body by acting as a vasodilator. This means it helps the blood vessels to widen, allowing more blood to flow around the body at any given time. This can not only aid in pretty much every function but also has various important roles in the brain and can be used to help us wake up in the morning!

Vitamin D

Vitamin D should be considered less a vitamin and more a 'master hormone'. Among other things,
vitamin D aids in the production of testosterone which helps boost muscle mass, weight loss, energy levels, libido and more! Vitamin D is mainly produced in the body in response to exposure to sunlight, though it can also be found in eggs. A recent study found that vitamin D is needed for the mitochondria in the cells to regenerate after exertion.

CoQ10: CoQ10 is another substance that can improve cellular energy by improving mitochondrial efficiency. Another is PQQ. These have been shown to improve not only athletic performance but also brain power.

Resveratrol

Resveratrol is one of the most powerful antioxidants we can get from the diet and is often thought of as being one of the most important aspects of the 'Mediterranean Diet'. The Mediterranean Diet is a diet that consists of foods similar to hot European countries and the logic behind this is that these cultures statistically enjoy longer lifespan and lower incidences of heart disease (this was especially surprising back when we thought that saturated fats cause heart problems!) Resveratrol is not only a potent antioxidant in its own right but also improves mitochondrial performance in a way that reduces the formation of free radicals in the first place. It has been shown to greatly extend the lifespan of rats in laboratory settings in a manner similar to calorie restriction

Glutathione

Glutathione is often described as the body's 'master antioxidant'. This molecule helps to detoxify the cells and combat free radicals and can unlock the full potential of all the other antioxidants in your system. In fact, without adequate levels of glutathione, your body cannot make full use of any other antioxidants from your diet. Vitamin C, fish, resveratrol and more all become much more potent when combined with a supply of Glutathione.

Calcium

Calcium is one of the minerals most responsible for strengthening the bones and connective tissue. It needs a good supply of magnesium and vitamin D for you to get the most of it.

Vitamin B

Vitamin B complex vitamins include B6, B12, thiamine, folate and riboflavin. These vitamins can be used for a number of things but are particularly powerful for converting protein and sugar into energy and producing red blood cells. In other words, adding vitamin B to your diet will improve energy metabolism and help you to wake up feeling refreshed!

Vitamin C

Vitamin C is a powerful antioxidant that is well known for helping to fend off all manner of diseases too by strengthening the immune system. It also happens to help with the production of serotonin thereby boosting the mood.

Protein

Protein is what we get from meat and it's where we get the 'amino acids' our bodies need. Amino acids are used when repairing skin and bone and for building muscle but they come in a range of different shapes and sizes.

To grow as much muscle as possible, the recommendation is that we get around 1 gram of protein for every one pound of body weight! Of course this advice is aimed at bodybuilders and athletes and wouldn't apply to the Average Joe. but it shows what a key role protein plays in our body composition.

What's also important to bear in mind is that there is more than one 'type' of amino acid. Actually, there are currently thought to be 20 amino acids, with nine of these only being available through the body. If you don't get all of these amino acids from your diet, then certain important repair jobs around your body will not get carried out. Seeing as most sources of protein only contain certain combinations of amino acids, it's generally important to make sure your diet contains a variety of different types of plants, fish, dairy and meats.

And it gets more complicated than that too – as protein sources also vary in their 'availability'. Depending on the ratio of essential to non-essential amino acids, the presence of branched-chain amino acids and other factors, certain proteins will be easier for the body to use than others.

With the best will in the world, animal sources are always superior to plant sources of protein. Why? Because animals are closer to us in structure. When you consume animal protein – like whey, egg, chicken or beef – you are consuming muscle and fat and skin and these are all things the body can use. Even soy protein is less effective and may also lower testosterone and increase oestrogen.

You also need to think about the vitamins and minerals you're getting and how you're keeping them in your diet. Because vitamins, minerals and other micronutrients can do all kinds of incredible things for your health.

In fact, many of the individual nutrients in our food are now sold as supplements for a variety of athletes. Never buy these supplements because that getting these nutrients from the diet is much easier, cheaper and more effective. When you get fat soluble minerals and vitamins from avocado instead of a tablet for instance, you also get that all-important saturated fat that helps you to absorb it. Meanwhile, getting iron from spinach versus a tablet means you're less likely to suffer with stomach problems. Moreover, it's simply impossible to add all of the different vitamins and minerals in your diet manually. It might sound like a good idea to take three different supplements every day to try and boost your energy levels but ask yourself: are you going to do this every single day? For the rest of your life??

On the other hand though, if you can get all this nutrition from your diet, then simply by eating a very balanced selection of different foods, you'll find that you're able to get an incredible range of different benefits. And the variety itself will also provide further advantages. A lot of the nutrients you'll get from a balanced diet are things we don't even know about yet – so you couldn't get them from supplementation even if you tried!

Fiber

Fiber may also play an important role in excess weight issues caused by hypothyroidism. Adult men generally need around 38 grams of fiber daily, while women need about 25 grams.

One type of fiber supplement is psyllium and those taking this supplement are less likely to consume fat and generally feel full a lot more quickly. Among the many kinds of fiber, there are even some that can help in insulin metabolism and this is proven to be especially useful for people who have a few extra pounds around the middle of their body.

Abdominal weight gain often leads to increasing insulin levels and this starts the whole metabolic syndrome going into overdrive, so this can be at least partially prevented by consuming the recommended amounts of fiber on a daily basis.

Body Detoxification
What Is Body Detoxification?

Body detoxification concentrates on cleaning out your digestive system, usually by drinking a solution that is made to clear out your intestines and give the organs in your digestive system a boost. Although it may sound like a surgical procedure, body detoxification only involves drinking and then going to the bathroom. That is all there is to the procedure. It works to make sure that your digestive system is healthy.

When your digestive system is in good working order, your whole body sings. If your digestive system is not healthy, then your whole body suffers. In order to have a healthy body, you must have a healthy digestive system.

But your digestive system is the catch all for all of the toxins that you take into your body. Even if you are a healthy person who does not smoke, does not drink and eats only organic foods, you are still taking in toxins. They are in the air that your breath, the water that you drink and well, just about everywhere. These toxins linger in the body and find their way to the digestive system.

The digestive system is comprised of organs such as the liver, pancreas, kidneys and intestines. Foods usually enter the digestive system through the stomach and are then passed for processing through the digestive tract. Some foods and drinks that you take in make the kidneys and pancreas work overtime in processing them. All of the organs in the digestive system have a job to do in order to keep your body running healthy. Once food and drink is processed in the system, it is then eliminated by way of waste. Liquids are eliminated by urine and solid waste is eliminated through the intestines as feces.

In some cases, foods can end up getting stuck in the intestines. There are cases where people have had elements in their intestines for 10 years! In addition, the organs also take a beating when it comes to getting rid of toxins as well as some foods that can be difficult for these organs to process. Simple carbohydrates, for example, are very hard on the kidneys and pancreas as well as the liver as they tend to pass through quickly and make these organs work overtime.

Toxins in the air that you breathe enter the system through the circulatory system that brings blood to and from the organs. When you smoke, for example, the smoke is absorbed into your bloodstream and carried throughout your body. This negatively affects the digestive system. Even second hand smoke will take its toll.

Your skin is your biggest organ and when you take a bath or shower using chemicals as are featured in shampoo and soap, you are absorbing toxins into your skin. When you breathe in air, you take the toxins into your lungs. It is impossible to live your life toxin free, although a good many people try. You are going to eventually go out and pick up germs that are in the air. It is inevitable that you will come into contact with toxins unless you decide to live your life in a plastic bubble.

Body detoxification clears the body of all of the toxins and foods that sit in the digestive system. Not only is it a good way to get the poisons out of your body, but it also works well when it comes to losing weight. Most people find that they can take off quite a few pounds simply by using body detoxification.

Drinking body detoxification fluid is similar to taking a barium enema, except you do not have to drink as much and it tastes much better. A barium enema completely clears out your intestines and is usually given to those who are having tests done on their colon or other digestive organs. This eliminates all of the waste from the body and makes you feel lighter. Not only can it get rid of toxins, but it can get rid of any waste that is lingering in your intestines.

Drinking the body detoxification formula is one of the first steps towards being healthier. You should also take proper precautions when it comes to your health and eat right, exercise and avoid bad habits. Body detoxification should be seen as a way to enhance your health, help you lose weight and keep your digestive system healthy. Good body detoxification will also fill your body with the nutrients that you may be lacking so that you stay healthy as well.

Detoxification For Weight Loss

If you are trying to lose weight, you may want to try body detoxification. This will get rid of the waste in your body and you will feel much lighter. Many people who are looking for a way to lose weight opt for body detoxification. body detoxification is one of the healthiest ways to lose weight.

Because you tend to store waste in your intestines, you may end up feeling bloated and retaining weight. body detoxification eliminates the waste from your body and makes you feel lighter instantly. That being said, body detoxification is not a laxative. It is a natural way to eliminate waste from your system that leads to weight loss.

Get Rid Of Toxins

A lot of the people are using body detoxification to rid themselves of toxins in which they imbibe on a regular basis. You can get rid your body of toxins by using a body cleanse system. This will work towards keeping your body clean and free from poisons that are in what you consume as well as what you breathe. If you smoke, drink or do not always eat a healthy diet, you can use body detoxification as a way to stay healthier and rid your body of toxins. While body detoxification should not be a substitute for practicing good health, it can help alleviate the problems that come with taking in toxins.

Just about everyone comes into contact with toxins. Ridding the body of toxins by using body detoxification is not only good for the digestive system, but also good for overall health.

Detoxification for Healthy Digestive System

Remember, your digestive system and its health is vital to the overall health of your body. Colon cancer, which is cancer of the small intestine, is the number 3 cancer killer in the United States. Colon cancer is the result of polyps in the colon. These polyps often result due to waste remaining in the colon. body detoxification gets rid of the waste in the body and keeps the colon clean. On top of that, many body detoxification formulas have herbs, vitamins and minerals in them that can help the body detoxify the digestive system and can feed the organs with nutrients that are needed to keep it cleansed. Many people use body detoxification as a way to maintain a healthy digestive system.

With natural body detoxification supplies, the body is fed a series of nutrients that not only end up helping the digestive system, but the rest of the body. The digestive organs send nutrients back through the body and to the heart, brain and other vital organs. body detoxification cleanse the entire body through the digestive organs.

Body detoxification is the safe way to lose weight fast. Instead of taking weight loss pills that often contain illegal pharmaceutical ingredients, you can take off the weight with a body detoxification system. You can create your own body detoxification by mixing water with ingredients such as lemon and pepper that will cleanse out your system. There are also commercial brands of weight loss body detoxification products that you can purchase.

Using the body detoxification systems to lose weight is safer than diet drinks that act as laxatives and contain chemicals. When you are looking for a body detoxification solution to help you lose weight, look for one that has all natural ingredients instead of one that is filled with chemicals as this will not only help you lose weight, but will also be healthier for your body.

Body detoxification not only rids your body of impurities that are found in the air, foods and drinks but it also can get rid your body of ailments. If you are trying to get over a cold, have stress or physical ailments, you will be surprised at how the body detoxification works to detoxify your system and make you feel better.

Exercise is also essential for body detoxification. You should perform cardiovascular exercises that will work up a sweat as well as relaxing exercises, such as yoga, to eliminate stress. Many people today complain of stress over work, home or money. Stress can play havoc on your body and natural body detoxification should try to eliminate stress as much as possible. Exercise is a natural way to not only get in shape and burn calories, but also to sweat out toxins.

Home Made Detoxifiers
Home Made Remedies for detoxification

You can easily make your own home made remedies that are ideal for home body detoxification. I will explore the different remedies that you can use.

Mother of all Detoxifier

i called this detoxifier " mother of all detoxifier" because this detoxifier will detoxify whole body and by using this detoxifier you will definitely lose weight

Ginger Juice – 1 cup

Garlic Juice – 1 cup

Lemon Juice – 1 cup

Apple Cider Vinegar – 1 cup

Organic Honey – 3 cup

Take ginger juice, garlic juice, lemon juice and vinegar in a sauce pan and cook on medium flame for 30 mins. Keep mixing.

now let it cool completely.

Now Add 3 cups of honey and mix well.

fill in clean bottle and store in fridge, you can store it for 30 days

Other detoxifiers
Detoxifier One

Lemon Pepper Cleanser

Both lemon and pepper combined will work well to zip through the body as a cleanser. Lemon pepper cleanser is one of the easiest and effective home cleansing remedies.

Detoxifier One – lemon pepper

8 Ounces of Water

2 Teaspoons of lemon zest

½ Teaspoon of black pepper

Combine the water and the other ingredients and drink it down. After you are finished drinking the solution, drink two 8 ounce glasses of water. This will help flush the solution into your system. Lemon pepper cleanser is good for the colon and entire digestive system.

For best results, use fresh ground black pepper and fresh lemon zest from a fresh lemon.

Alternate use - You can omit the black pepper and add one teaspoon of fresh lemon juice to the mix

Detoxifier Two

Italian body detoxifier
 8 Ounces of Water
1 Teaspoon of flaxseed oil
1 Teaspoon of Basil
1 Teaspoon of Oregano
½ Teaspoon of Garlic

Combine all of the ingredients with the water and drink it. After drinking, wait five minutes for the solution to settle and then drink two more glasses of water. This acts as a detoxifier for the entire body and is good for both the digestive system as well as the circulatory system.
For best results, use fresh herbs and garlic.
Alternate use - You can substitute Rosemary for Basil.

Detoxifier Three

Berry Detox
6 Ounces of Water
2 Ounces of Pure Acai Berry Juice
½ Cup Blueberries
4 Fresh Strawberries

Put all of the ingredients in the blender and mix them together. Drink them and follow the solution with an 8 ounce glass of purified water. This is a detoxifier that is loaded with antioxidants and purifiers.
For best results, use only fresh ingredients.
Alternate use - Substitute ½ cup of blueberries for the strawberries.

Detoxifier Four

Tropical Detox
1 Banana
1 cup unsweetened, plain yogurt
 ½ cup pure orange juice
½ cup pure pineapple juice

Put all ingredients into a blender and the mix them. This will be more like a shake than a traditional drink but works well to cleanse out the digestive tract as well as provide essential nutrients. This works slower than other body detoxifiers but is healthy for the colon as well as the heart and immune system.
For best results - Use only fresh ingredients and pure juices
Alternative - You can 1 cup of orange juice instead of half and half of pineapple juice and orange juice.

Detoxifier Five

Energizing Cleanse
 8 Ounces of Water
 1 Teaspoon of Maca Root
1 Teaspoon of Ginseng
1 Teaspoon of Acai powder

You may have to use pestle and mortar to break up the roots, especially if they are fresh, as they should be. You can purchase liquid Ginseng, although you are better off to purchase capsule forms. Grind up the dry ingredients, mix them with the Acai powder and then add them to the water. Drink down the mixture and then drink another glass of water.

This will not only give you energy to spare, but will also work towards detoxifying your digestive and circulatory system. If you are looking for a way to energize your body, this will do it.

You can purchase the supplements in any health food store or even online. Make sure that they are pure supplements and not just chemically reproduced. Ginseng is often available in "energy drinks" in stores - avoid that and get the actual product.

Detoxifier Six

Colon Cleanse Diet
8 Ounces of Water
1 Teaspoon of FlaxSeed Oil
1 Teaspoon of FRESH ginger
1 Teaspoon of Grape seed oil
1 Package of green tea

This is a body detoxifier that works well as a colon cleanser. Add the ingredients together before adding to the water. You may need to use the mortar and pestle to grind up the ginger if you do not have a food processor. You want only to use fresh ginger for this cleanse. Open up the package of green tea and dump it into the mix.
Mix everything with the water and then drink. Follow it with two glasses of water. This is a good weight loss detoxifier that you can make right from products that you purchase at the supermarket.
For best results, Use only fresh ingredients that are pure
Alternate use - Use a green tea capsule and grind it up with the mortar and pestle.

Detoxifier Seven

Cinnamon Spice
1 cup of brewed green tea
1 teaspoon of honey
½ teaspoon of cinnamon

After you have brewed the green tea, add the cinnamon and the honey to the mixture and drink it hot. This is a pleasant tasting drink and will not only relax you, but will also cleanse out your body and help your heart.
For best results - Use fresh ground cinnamon

Detoxifier Eight

Kidney Cleansing
8 Ounces of Water
½ Cup pure cranberry juice
¼ Cup pure Acai juice
3 Teaspoons orange juice

Mix the ingredients together and add them to the water. Drink it down and then drink two more 8 ounce glasses of water. This will help clean out your urinary tract and clear up urinary tract infections.
For best results - Use only pure ingredients and 100 percent pure orange juice

Detoxifier Nine

Lavender Cleansing
8 Ounces of Water
1 Teaspoon of pure Lavender oil
1 Teaspoon of FlaxSeed oil

Mix the oils with the water and drink. Consume another glass of water after to flush down the mixture. This is a total body cleanse and will detoxify all parts of your body.
Warning - Use only pure Lavender oil. Essential oils, with the exception of a few, are not made for ingestion Lavender oil is an exception, but it must be pure.

Detoxifier Ten

Tropical Delight
 Ice Cubes made from purified water
½ Banana
1 Teaspoon of Flax Seed Oil
½ Cup orange juice
¼ Cup Acai juice
2 Teaspoons of Lemon juice (pure)
Mix all of the ingredients together in a blender. Add enough ice cubes to fill the blender and then purifier. Drink the entire amount of the potion. This is a detoxifier for the body and can also substitute as a meal if you are trying to lose weight.

Detoxifier Eleven

Veggie Cleanser
1 Fresh Carrot, peeled
2 Crowns of Broccoli
1 Teaspoon of Omega Fish Oil
1 Teaspoon Flax Seed Oil
Ice Cubes

You need a food processor for this recipe, although it certainly cleans out the system and works wonders on the digestive system. You have to pulverize the vegetables so that they are like mush and then add the ice cubes and oils to the mix. Mix well and then consume the entire amount. Follow with a glass of purified water.

This is a safe and healthy drink that can be consumed on a healthy basis. It can also be used as a substitute for a meal if you are dieting.

Detoxifier Twelve

Vitamin Cleanser
1 Cup Green Tea - Hot
1 Capsule of Vitamin D
1 Capsule of Vitamin A
1 Capsule of Vitamin K
½ Teaspoon of Cinnamon

Grind up the capsules in a mortar and then add them to the hot tea so that they dissolve. Then add the cinnamon to the mix. Drink it down. This will add vitamins and nutrients to your body that you may be lacking. It is good for eliminating stress, depression and also healthy for the heart.

All of the ingredients for these body detoxifiers can be found at your local grocery store or health food store. You need to make sure that you are purchasing pure ingredients and not those made from synthetics

Green tea is one of the key components when it comes to weight loss through body detoxification. Green tea acts like a diuretic and can help you lose weight quicker. You should drink green tea without sugar in order to get the effects. Drink plenty of green tea a day and you will find that you are taking off the pounds. Green tea can also be taken in tablet form if you dislike the taste.

Cranberry also works as a diuretic and can help you lose weight through body detoxification. Cranberry should be used in tablet form as the juice drinks that you purchase in the grocery store are loaded with sugar. Cranberry will also help clean out your urinary tract.

Water It is important that you drink plenty of water when you are body detoxifying to lose weight. You never want to diet without supplementing yourself with water. By drinking 8 glasses of water a day and using a good, natural body detoxifier, you will take off weight quicker than dieting alone.

Exercising

Exercising and dieting are two things that go hand in hand. If you just diet without exercising, you may not see any result at all because you are not losing calories fast enough in your diet. Also if you do manage to lose weight without dieting, you would look thin and frail as you lose your fat. So it is better to exercise to keep your body fit while you diet. There are also other reasons to exercise.

A recent survey showed that seven out of ten adults do not exercise regularly and close to four out of ten are not physically active. If you do not exercise, then you will risk getting stroke, diabetes and heart disease. This has led to death for about 300 000 people.

Before you start exercising, you should consult a physician. This is to know your current body condition and see if you would risk injuries if you perform tiring exercise activities. When you first start out exercising, do it slowly. First start off with only 10 minutes which then is increase to 20 minutes then to 30 minutes and so on and so forth over the period of months. This will help avoid your body to feel very sore after each work out and decrease any injury risk.

You should at least do 30 minutes or more of moderate cardiovascular activities each day. You do not have to do all 30 minutes together; it can be even short bouts of intermittent activities. Then twice a week, do exercise that would train your muscles. You can incorporate this physical exercise into your daily life. For example, take the stairs to the office instead of the elevator; go for a jog during your lunch time or park further away from your work place.

If you feel this is too much of a chore, why not try to make your leisure time more active. Instead of sitting at home only, ask your family out for a bicycle ride, join a rock climbing club or just stroll the park every evening.

Pick out exercising activities that you would enjoy to do, find it satisfying and gives you a feeling of accomplishment. A successful run will motivate you more to be physically active. Make it easy for you to be active by picking exercise that is easier accessible so you will not be unmotivated every time you want to perform your exercise. Lastly, pick out exercise that is compatible with your body and current age.

Types Of Exercises

First of all, you need to know that there are three kinds of exercise plans which are available and all three of them have different advantages for your physical health.

Exercise To Improve Bone and Muscle Strength

These exercises are also called strength and resistance training. Most of the people take body building as strength and resistance increasing exercise but you need to know that body building is another category of exercise in which the primary goal of the person is to enhance muscle growth.

You can add some weight lifting and body building in your fat burning and weight control plan but you should do it to an extent where your body can bear it without any problem. If you over tried this exercise then, your whole body can be a mess. I have seen people joining gyms and doing hard exercise just by watching other people doing it. This is not the way to go instead consult your trainer personally and ask him about appropriate exercises which can fit in your needs. If your weight is under control and you need just light exercise to keep your healthy system going then, you do not need to lift heavy weights.

Flexibility Increasing Exercises

Second type of exercise plan can be to increase your flexibility and in more common terms you can say that if you used to have pain in your arms, legs, lower back, neck and other similar areas of your body then, you need to make your body more flexible. Flexibility will increase resistance and you will be able to cope with more difficult positions and postures easily. You have to go through different postures in daily life for example if you work in an office then, you can be given an uncomfortable chair at times or you may be given some work in which you have to concentrate hard on computer screen and you cannot rest your back with chair. In these situations, if you do not have any flexibility in your body then, it will create problems but regular flexibility exercises which will not take more than 10-15 minutes of your time, will increase this flexibility and will make you feel better and active.

Cardiovascular Exercise

Cardio means heart and vascular means the vessels of blood and this whole phrase means that these exercises improve the functionality of your lungs and make the use of oxygen more effective and rectify any heart problems which you can have. These exercises are little time consuming and should be properly learned from your doctor or trainer. Most of the times, people who already have got some heart problem perform these kinds of exercises to avoid any future problems.

Finding Exercises To Be Done At Home

A major change has been observed in the tendency of workout freaks, which is changing their exercise locale from gyms to home. Reason being, the soaring membership prices and binding contracts. As a result, they have started to opt for home fitness programs.

Finding exercises to be done at home is not a complex job, rather a much more convenient option. There are many great cardio exercises which can be done without much cost to the users. The main money spent is in a good pair of walking, jogging or aerobic shoe, depending on the kind of activity desired. Besides, a jumping rope is also a great addition for skipping at home because it provides users added alternatives of aerobic workouts that can include rapid work interval training. One can do it while watching TV or may be by playing music alongside. One should jump for a duration of thirty seconds to a minute as fast as possible and rest in between for sometime before starting again. You can always perform it during ad commercials and watch the rest of your show calming your body. Today, video and DVD market is flooded with

exercise, aerobics and yoga CDs and DVDs which can be purchased for a favorable fitness exercise regime to start at home.

This gives more alternatives to people in case jogging or walking becomes mundane or if the weather does not allow you to go outside and run. Running and walking can actually become all the more interesting if done with a partner, provided no chit-chat and gossip hours begin and win over your fitness schedule. '

Varying the ground of the running or walking area can also add change to the daily workout process. Remember, it is very essential that you enjoy what you do to keep yourself fit if you actually want to feel the change in your health and body. Besides, age does matter while selecting the kind of workout that you do. An adult person may be capable of losing weight using particular equipments and build muscles as well, but an elderly may not just get the same results from the same regimen. It is simply because of the quality of performance and not the utilization the expensive and similar machines. Thu, it's advisable that you always choose a kind of fitness regimen that goes well with your body, age and needs keeping the various health constraints that age brings along.

Exercises At Home
Exercises that you can perform at home

Leaving you with no excuses of not finding the right type of exercises that you can do at home, here is a list of the appropriate home fitness based program exercises for you-

These exercises can be performed by using easy drills at home and employing minimal

equipments which you can get from around your house.

For upper body you can do chair dips, lateral raises, push-ups, chin ups and bent

over row. For core exercises you can do dead lift, sit ups and Side Bridge.

For lower body you can opt for step ups, wall squat, bucket squats and lunges.

Prior to starting these exercises you must warm up yourself for minimum of five minutes by jogging or brisk walk around the block or by skipping on the spot. You must perform multiple sets of the exercises mentioned above depending upon your endurance level and requirement. Also, taking intervals in between is equally essential. You can combine two exercises that use diverse muscle groups alternating between two things that provide each muscle group some rest while you perform another.

To get the best results, perform these workouts at least three times a week, with no less than a day between exercises for sufficient recovery. You must always strive to increase the intensity or load and to increase your fitness growth. Once your fitness improves, you can undergo this routine without bothering much and start with a more superior program. Use your creativity and find more things to use for working out at home.

Using buckets, filled with the amount of water you want can be employed for squats and step-ups.

Filling up milk bottles with 2 liter water makes it equivalent to a 2 kg weight to be used

for overhead triceps extension, bicep curls and bent over rows.

Shopping bags and backpack filled with items can be used for lunges, step-ups and squats. Utilizing bricks by breaking them in half in case of lower weight is appropriate for pushups, bench press, lateral raises and front raise.

Then comes the age old forms of exercises that come under the practice of yoga asana. A lot of people not just perform these exercises for the sole aim of relieving mental stress but to get and stay fit as well. If you look at the fitness regimens of every famous celebrity today including the big names like Jennifer Aniston, Drew Barrymore, it is yoga that has worked wonders on their body to get the envious figure every girl wants. Not only women, even men have also started incorporating this form of fitness to build up muscles using their own body weight. This is the most natural way of dealing with your body and respecting it as well.

Getting Physical

Quick fact: Remember what we mentioned before? There are approximately 3,500 calories per pound of fat?

That means that you need to burn 3,500 calories to lose one pound of fat.

Makes you think twice before eating a hamburger with the fries doesn't it? especially when you put it into perspective with the amount of exercise you have to do to burn it off. That always makes me think twice before reaching for the tub of ice cream because I think how much I'll have to sweat and burn to get rid of it.

But don't think for a second that you need to be like those Biggest Loser Guys on television where they lose an unrealistic 10 to 15 pounds per week.

Who has the time to exercise for 6 to 7 hours per day? Not me and I'm pretty sure neither do you. I wouldn't recommend this method of weight loss; it's simply not realistic for the general population to follow when you have a fulltime job and family to worry about. Great if you can hole yourself up for 12 weeks with a personal trainer, all of the latest cutting edge technology equipment and with the entire world watching you're every move, who wouldn't succeed?

Please don't think that because you are not losing 5 pounds per week
that you're failing your program or that it's not working.
Don't compare your results to these types of shows as the conditions they lose the weight under are extreme.
A recent study revealed that if you give someone a good enough reason to lose weight, they will. 25 overweight participants had pictures taken of them wearing nothing more than their underwear revealing of all their lumps, bumps and jiggly bits.
The challenge for the group was for everyone to lose at least 10 pounds in the next month or run the risk of having their picture published on the front page of the highest publication newspaper. 30 days later, how successful do you think the experiment was?
100% success rate and why wouldn't it be? If you were faced with humiliation you would do anything to avoid the pain of it. Same thing with the Biggest Loser contestants, not only is money a motivating factor but who wants to look like a failure in front of the world?
Wouldn't it make you want to work just that little bit harder? you bet it would.

So please don't put yourself under unrealistic pressure to match pound for pound what these contestants are losing. I recall once reading a weight loss forum post where a woman was so depressed having only had lost 3 pounds in one week compared to her favorite female contestant who had lost 8 pounds. It derailed her diet because she couldn't keep up, she thought she wasn't working hard enough which left her disheartened and feeling like she failed.

A pound of fat is a pound of fat no matter how you look at it; it's a tiny miraculous achievement that adds up to your bigger goal. Whether you lose 1 pound, 3 pounds or zero pounds in a given week shouldn't throw you from your overall goal because you need to remember everyone is different and will lose weight at different rates. Even if you don't lose any weight in one week doesn't mean you are not making progress. Remember that weight fluctuations will happen and if your weight seems like it's not budging fast enough, I'm sure your clothes will prove differently.

Any weight loss is great. Just keep with it.

The thought makes most people cringe but don't worry, we aren't going to ask you to go out and spend hours in the gym working off your weight one mile at a time on the treadmill.

Instead you're going to get a no nonsense approach to exercise anyone can do despite your current level of fitness.

Exercise in your life

Ok, let's start the show by busting a myth or two along the way. Contrary to popular belief sneaking in a little housework during commercial breaks doesn't cut the mustard. It won't be enough to lose the excess pounds you gained over the years.

For exercise to be of any long term benefit you have to raise your heart rate for at least 30 minutes at a time for at least 3 or more times per week.

Would you believe that some people don't consider walking around the neighborhood or up stairs as significant exercise? It may be low impact but it is better than doing no exercise at all and whether you realize it or not still burns calories.

When you think of exercise what images do you conjure in your mind?

Is it of sweaty bodies squeezed into a tiny spaces jumping to pounding music? Exercise doesn't have to be a torture; it can be enjoyable especially if shared with your family of friends. Exercise can be going for a walk, chasing after your children, mowing and raking the lawn. Anything that gets your heart rate up for an extended period of time is considered exercise.

Benefits Of Exercise

Exercise And Its Far Reaching Benefits

Exercise, why even do it? Whether you like it or not it's the only way we can burn the excess stores of energy we have accumulated over the years, otherwise known as fat. Our body has stored it but thankfully it can get rid of it too and in order to do that, you've got to move. It's the only way your lean muscle tissue can grab the surrounding fat to burn as energy.

Long after your exercise session whether it be walking, running, swimming, biking, etc, your metabolism continues to burn calories even when you are at rest. The effects of exercise can be experienced long after the actual exercise itself. This is evident in that you sweat a little easier which means your body is behaving like a fat burning furnace, any exercise you do after that point just turbo charges the exercise you've already done and burns extra calories.

Exercise has so many benefits

Exercise prolongs your life and keeps your heart healthy. Don't forget that the heart itself is a muscle and needs exercise too. That's why you should resist taking the easy way by going to those spas that claim you can lose weight by doing nothing or than sweating. Sure you lose inches but they find their way like a magnet back onto your body with the next glass of water you drink. Resist gimmicks, if it sounds too good to be true it probably is. Exercise, get your heart rate going, it's the best thing you can do for yourself and your heart will thank you for it.

Exercise also releases your body's natural feel good chemicals known as endorphins (a combination of the words endogenous and morphine) which naturally relieve stress. Endorphins are thought to be as powerful as morphine yet they are not addictive and are produced naturally within the body. They are also the body's natural pain relief.

Exercise has so many additional benefits including increased agility and stamina, improved memory and reaction time, increase bone density, keeps your arteries supple and flexible for blood to flow through. Reduces the risk of heart attack and stroke. Stronger immune system and deeper, restful sleep.

Exercise helps you to live longer, people who do 30 to 60 minutes of exercise 3 or more times per week will generally live longer than those who don't.

I don't know about you but that builds a pretty strong case in favor of exercise.

Here are some daily calorie burning activities you can do along with the value of calories burned associated with it.

Note – before embarking on any exercise program it is highly recommended that you first consult your physician to assess your current physical state.

Calories Burned Chart

Which workout burn how much calories

Note – these are the average figures for a 185 pound individual, results will vary according to weight. If you are a little heavier you will burn more calories than the figures presented below. These figures are based upon 60 minutes of activity.

- Ironing – 189 calories
- Washing dishes – 189 calories
- Cooking – 222 calories
- Carpentry – 300 calories
- Lawn raking – 333 calories
- Mopping – 377 calories
- Housework– 390 calories
- Gardening – 455 calories
- Wood Chopping – 511 calories
- Furniture rearranging – 555

Exercise as you can see comes in many forms not only are there practical and useful applications but you also get the added benefit of it improving your health.

However if you are serious about losing weight you have to step up your efforts a little more, these everyday household activities are great for getting exercise but as you know in order to lose even a pound of fat you need to lose 3,500 calories. It would take a lot of furniture moving and gardening for you to get to that point.

To get to the stage where you will lose weight on a consistent basis you need to add extra exercise to your routine.

Let's start small because these are activities that can boost your level of fat burning that little bit extra.

These activities aren't too strenuous but can help the weight come off faster.

Light Exercise

This is achievable for most people no matter what your fitness level and will kick your weight loss up a notch.

Note – these are the average figures for a 185 pound individual, results will vary according to weight. If you are a little heavier you will burn more calories than the figures presented below. These figures are based upon 60 minutes of activity.

- An hour's worth of Yoga stretching – 350 calories
- A relaxing bike ride for one hour – 350 calories
- Running around with your children – 350 calories
- Lawn mowing – 366 calories
- Basketball (shooting hoops) – 377 calories
- Pilates – 433 calories
- Walking (4 miles per hour) – 433 calories
- Game of golf – 480 calories
- Snow shoveling – 511 calories
- Walking up stairs – 577 calories
- Stationary bike – 588 calories
- Walking on a treadmill or jogging – 588 calories
- Low intensity jump rope – 700 calories

Light exercise is fantastic because it can be easily incorporated into our daily lives and will be the exercise most people, especially when starting off on a weight loss program will be able to do.

Once the weight starts to come off and you gain a little more confidence you no doubt will be able to introduce more rigorous exercise into your regime. When you feel within yourself your fitness level increasing you might want to try some moderate exercise.

Moderate Exercise

Here are some examples of moderate exercise. Again these figures are representative of a 185 pound person. If you weigh more than this your calorie expenditure will be much higher. These figures are based upon 60 minutes of activity.

- Low impact Aerobics – 431 calories
- Hiking – 499 calories
- Swimming (moderate) – 511 calories
- Hiking (medium terrain) – 520 calories
- Jogging – 588 calories
- Step Aerobics – 588 calories
- Basketball officiating – 588 calories
- Jogging – 600 calories
- Rollerblading – 600 calories
- Repelling – 677 calories
- Game of Ice hockey – 700 calories
- Press-ups/sit-ups – 700 calories
- Mountain Biking – 710 calories
- Running (5 miles per hour) – 710 calories
- Ski Machine – 810 calories
- Rowing machine (minimal effort) – 820 calories
- Jump rope (moderate effort) – 860 calories

If you want to take your weight loss to newfound levels you can introduce more intense exercise to your routine known as heavy exercise. Not only will it build more fat stripping lean muscle tissue but it will make your body both inside and out stronger than ever.

Heavy Exercise

These exercises are the same as above but with the difference of increased intensity level.

Remember that if you have been sedentary for quite some time, you may want to build up to these activities by trying the lower intensity alternatives first.

Again these figures are representative of a 185 pound person. If you weigh more than this your calorie expenditure will be much higher. These figures are based upon 60 minutes of activity.

- Step Aerobics (high impact) – 888 calories
- Rock Climbing – 921 calories
- Basketball Full Court – 921 calories
- Bikram Yoga – 950 calories
- Elliptical Trainer – 955 calories
- Swimming (butterfly stroke) – 1,000 calories
- Handball – 1,010 calories
- A game of Squash – 1,040 calories
- Canoeing (above 6 mph) – 1,040 calories
- Jumping rope (high impact) – 1,040 calories
- Cross-country skiing (high impact) around 1,400 calories.
- Running (12 miles per hour) – 1,876 calories

Finding an exercise program that is right for you

There will only ever be 24 hours in a day and how we use those will have a huge impact on our weight loss success. I know it's not easy. With the crazy pace of our lives in the 21st century we are finding ourselves busier than we ever have before at any other time in history and as a result, we may find it difficult to incorporate exercise into our hectic schedules.

The reality will always be that if you want to have any success with your weight loss efforts you have to be able to exercise and make it as part of your new lifestyle.

But just because you will be adding exercise to your daily routine doesn't mean that you have to join a gym unless you really want to.

Even just watching a little less television and opting instead to go for a brisk walk can contribute to your weight loss. Playing with the kids and exerting yourself a little more will burn extra calories. Finding the balance that's right for you and the exercises that you can work into your lifestyle without turning your whole life upside down is the key to your success.

If you find it difficult to materialize the time during your day to exercise then simply take the times that you undertake any kind of physical activity and amp it up just a fraction more to burn the extra calories.

Use the time you play with the kids to increase activity levels. Instead of just playing with them why not bike ride with them or throw a ball around at the same time? You still get to spend quality time with the added benefit of ditching extra calories.

Get active, sign up for a sport whether it's tennis, football, baseball, swimming or aerobics this is a great way to lose weight and have fun at the same time while making new friends (what a great way to get support). Even making the time to do this once per week can contribute to your overall weight loss.

If you work in an office building why not opt to take the stairs? To build up your fitness you may even wish to go past your own level. Not only is this a great way of increasing your fitness level but it's also fantastic for incorporating into your daily schedule so you in essence made it part of your new lifestyle change without having to make too great a sacrifice. Before know it, it will have become such an integral part of your life that you won't be able to do without it

Try hiring exercise equipment for home. Why hire? So that you don't get bored from using the same piece of equipment day in and day out.

When hiring you can advance to more challenging and sophisticated equipment the more your fitness increases and you're not stuck with the same thing each day.

By hiring you can continually upgrade and take advantage of the latest cutting edge equipment. The beauty of exercise equipment is that you get to exercise anywhere you want and why not take the opportunity to do an hour long workout during your favorite show, that way you get to enjoy the show while doing something beneficial for yourself. Don't forget though as with anything in life you only get out what you put in. So if you're going to go to the trouble of hiring a piece of equipment, you have to use it.

Not enough hours in the day? We can't create extra time however we can use wisely the time that we do have. Why not try jumpstarting your day an hour earlier by doing some exercise? Why not walk the dog? Why not do an hour on the treadmill or an hour of yoga or Pilates?

Not only do you kick start your metabolism into action but you will continue to burn calories long throughout your day as a result of your early morning exercise efforts.

Any activities that you do such as housecleaning or vacuuming, sweeping and mowing the lawn, why not put more effort and intensity into it? This can make an impact on your weight loss efforts just by doing a little more.

Any form of exercise is good and the more you do it and increase the intensity level the more fat you will burn. Aim to start with three times per week then increase from there and you will notice the results. Not only will your energy levels increase but you will notice your body changing and your clothes fitting looser on your body.

Remember that exercise is not just for the here and now; it's a lifestyle change for life. Beyond just wanting to look good you are prolonging your life in the process and the benefits far outweigh sacrificing a little down time. Your health and life are worth it.

Now come to the most popular weight loss program if you follow that diet program with regular exercise, there is no way you gain your weight again and the only way to lose weight rapidly is called intermittent fasting

Intermittent fasting
What is intermittent fasting?

Intermittent fasting is becoming a popular choice among people who are trying to lose weight. However, it is also popular with many other people who want to take advantage of its health benefits.

intermittent fasting vs. Other diet plans

Essentially, intermittent fasting is an eating pattern rather than a normal diet.

Standard diets focus on what you eat. Dieters are limited to a certain number of calories or certain types of food. This leads dieters to constantly think about what they are and what they are not allowed to eat. Oily and sugary foods are absolutely prohibited. There is a strong emphasis on vegetables, fruits and meals low in fat and sugar. Those who follow this type of food often fantasize about treats and snacks. Although they can lose weight, they may find it difficult to stick to their long-term diet.

Intermittent fasting is different. It's more a lifestyle than a diet. This includes eating habits where you switch between fasting and eating windows. Unlike other diets, it doesn't focus on what you eat. Instead, it focuses on when you need to eat. Some dieters enjoy the greatest freedom it gives them. You can eat the food they enjoy without guilt. Many people also find that it fits better with their lifestyle.

Popular type of intermittent fasting

There are different types of intermittent fasting. Each has its own advantage. All of them follow the same principle of restricting food intake for a certain period of time. However, the length and distance between meal windows varies.

Perhaps the most popular IF method is the 16: 8 method. This includes an 8-hour meal window followed by 16 hours of fasting. Many people find this to be the most convenient option for them. If you skip breakfast or dinner, you can easily integrate it into your lifestyle.

Another popular IF option is the 24 hour fast. This is sometimes called the eat-stop-eat method. It's about eating a normal day, then avoiding the next 24 hours. Deviations between fasts can only be 24 hours or up to 72 hours.

The 5: 2 fasting method is also popular. This includes normal eating five days a week. On the other two consecutive days, the diet should limit its calorie intake to around 500 to 600 calories.

Some IF dieters choose the 20: 4 method. This involves concentrating all daily meals on a four-hour window. The dieter should not eat calories for the other 20 hours of the day.

There are various other types of fasting foods. Some people stick to a long fast of up to 48 or 36 hours. Others fast longer. If you want to try IF, you have to choose the right method for you.

Why intermittent fasting?
Why do people prefer intermittent fasting?

Unlike other types of diets, IF allows dieters to eat just about what they want. You can eat the sugary or fatty foods of your dreams. You can go out to eat and not worry about the calories. You don't have to eat foods you don't like. You don't have to feel like they're flying even things they like. It is easy to understand why this choice is so popular.

Not only that, but also intermittent fasting offers many more benefits than other types of nutrition. Yes, it promotes rapid weight loss. However, it also helps dieters to feel more focused and productive. This helps them to feel healthier and more energetic. Given the health benefits this type of diet brings, it's no wonder people prefer a normal diet.

Benefits of intermittent fasting
Weight Loss

Many people who fast sometimes do so to lose weight quickly. This type of diet has been proven to help you lose those pounds faster. There are many reasons why IF helps you lose weight.

It also reduces the number of calories you consume in 24 hours. By lowering insulin levels and increasing growth hormone levels, FI accelerates fat loss. It also facilitates the use of fats for energy.

It improves metabolic function for faster fat burning. Fasting for a short time has been shown to increase the metabolic rate by up to 14%. This means that you are burning morc calorics. Therefore, FI can cause weight loss of up to 8% over a period of 3 to 24 weeks. It is an impressive loss!

Those who try IF report a 7% reduction in their lower size. This indicates a loss of abdominal fat - the most harmful type of fat that leads to illness.

As a bonus, FI causes less muscle loss compared to a reduced calorie diet.

Repair cells

When you fast, the cells in your body begin to remove waste products. This is called "autophagy". In autophagy, the cells of the body are degraded. It also involves the metabolism of dysfunctional and broken proteins that have accumulated in cells over time.

What is the advantage of autophagy? Experts believe that it offers protection against the development of several diseases. These include Alzheimer's disease and cancer.

So if you fast sometimes, you may be able to protect yourself from the disease. As a result, you can live a longer, healthier life.

Improved brain function

If something is good for your body, it is often also good for your brain. Intermittent fasting is known to improve various metabolic characteristics. These are crucial for good brain health.

Intermittent fasting has been shown to reduce oxidative stress. It also reduces inflammation and lowers blood sugar. Not only that, it also reduces insulin resistance, as we have shown above. These are all key factors for improving brain function.

As an added benefit, animal studies have shown that FI can protect against brain damage caused by stroke.

All of this suggests that intermittent fasting has many benefits for brain health.

Reduced inflammation

Oxidative stress is known to be a key factor in chronic disease and aging. Oxidative stress is made up of free radicals, which are unstable molecules that react with other key molecules such as DNA and proteins. The result is damage to molecules that damage the body.

Several studies have been conducted to prove that IF can help improve your body's ability to resist oxidative stress. Other studies have also shown that fighting inflammation, which also triggers many common illnesses, can help.

16: 8 Intermittent fasting

If you want to try intermittent fasting, you can start with 16: 8 fasting. This method involves fasting for 16 hours and then eating for 8 hours. It is one of the most popular forms of this type of food.

If you want to start the 16: 8 fast, you must first select a dining room window. This 8 hour period can apply at any time of the day. Therefore, you can choose the right time that suits your preferences and lifestyle. Once you have chosen your preferred eight hours, you should limit your food intake to those hours.

How do you choose the right hours for you? Many people like a window from 12 p.m. to 8 p.m. Indeed, they can fast overnight, skip breakfast, and then enjoy lunch and dinner at regular times. You can even include healthy snacks in your diet.

For those who prefer to eat three meals a day, one is at 9 a.m. - The restoration window at 5 p.m. may be the best. This allows breakfast at 9 a.m., lunch at 12 p.m. and dinner early at 4 p.m.

Others prefer to wait until the beginning of the afternoon to break the fast and then have their last meal later before going to bed.

Whichever dining window you choose, make sure it fits your lifestyle. If you choose wrong, you cannot stick to your diet.

Plan healthy food

To maximize the benefits of the 16: 8 diet, you should eat as much healthy food as possible. If you eat nutritious food, you will not be hungry or craving unhealthy food. This will help you stick to your new way of eating for the long term.

While you can enjoy snacks and treats, you need to balance each meal with a variety of whole foods. Some of the best are:

• Fruits such as bananas, apples, oranges, pears, peaches and berries

• Vegetables such as tomatoes, green leafy vegetables, cucumbers, cauliflower and broccoli

• Whole grain products such as oats, rice, quinoa, buckwheat and barley

• Healthy fats such as coconut oil, avocados and olive oil

• Lean proteins like poultry, fish, seeds, nuts, eggs and legumes

Eating junk food can negate the benefits of this diet. Therefore, you should always keep unhealthy decisions to a minimum.

Choose calorie-free drinks

You can drink any of your favorite drinks during your meal window. At least within reasonable limits! If you drink several bottles of whole family size soda, you will probably not lose weight!

In your fasting window, you only have to consume non-caloric drinks. When you consume a calorie drink, you are essentially breaking your fast. It ruins your whole diet.

Water, green tea, unsweetened coffee and tea without milk are good choices. They also help you control your appetite and keep you hydrated until you break your fast.

Weekly schedule

Your 16: 8 weekly meal plan depends on the meal window you choose. Here are three examples of different times:

Plan to eat early

Mon	Tues	Wed	Thurs	Fri	Sat	Sun
8a.m. - breakfast	8a.m. - breakfast	8a.m. - breakfast	8a.m. - breakfast	8a.m. - breakfast	8a.m. - breakfast	8a.m. - breakfast
10a.m. snack	10a.m. snack	10a.m. snack	10a.m. snack	10a.m. snack	10a.m. snack	10a.m. snack
12 noon - lunch	12 noon - lunch	12 noon - lunch	12 noon - lunch	12 noon - lunch	12 noon - lunch	12 noon – lunch
Evening – calorie-free beverages	Evening – calorie-free beverages	Evening – calorie-free beverages	Evening – calorie-free beverages	Evening – calorie-free beverages	Evening – calorie-free beverages	Evening – calorie-free beverages

Average Eating Meal Plan

Mon	Tues	Wed	Thurs	Fri	Sat	Sun
9a.m. – calorie-free beverage	9a.m. – calorie-free beverage	9a.m. – calorie-free beverage	9a.m. – calorie-free beverage	9a.m. – calorie-free beverage	9a.m. – calorie-free beverage	9a.m. – calorie-free beverage
11a.m. - breakfast	11a.m. - breakfast	11a.m. - breakfast	11a.m. - breakfast	11a.m. - breakfast	11a.m. - breakfast	11a.m. - breakfast
2p.m. lunch	2p.m. lunch	2p.m. lunch	2p.m. lunch	2p.m. lunch	2p.m. lunch	2p.m. lunch
4p.m. snack	4p.m. snack	4p.m. snack	4p.m. snack	4p.m. snack	4p.m. snack	4p.m. snack
6p.m. dinner	6p.m. dinner	6p.m. dinner	6p.m. dinner	6p.m. dinner	6p.m. dinner	6p.m. dinner

Late Eating Meal Plan

Mon	Tues	Wed	Thurs	Fri	Sat	Sun
11a.m. – calorie-free beverage	11a.m. – calorie-free beverage	11a.m. – calorie-free beverage	11a.m. – calorie-free beverage	11a.m. – calorie-free beverage	11a.m. – calorie-free beverage	11a.m. – calorie-free beverage
1p.m. snack	1p.m. snack	1p.m. snack	1p.m. snack	1p.m. snack	1p.m. snack	1p.m. snack
4p.m. lunch	4p.m. lunch	4p.m. lunch	4p.m. lunch	4p.m. lunch	4p.m. lunch	4p.m. lunch
6p.m. snack	6p.m. snack	6p.m. snack	6p.m. snack	6p.m. snack	6p.m. snack	6p.m. snack
9p.m. dinner	9p.m. dinner	9p.m. dinner	9p.m. dinner	9p.m. dinner	9p.m. dinner	9p.m. dinner

Exercise and intermittent fasting

Maximize your intermittent fasting results.

Some research shows that there are additional benefits to exercising while fasting. There is an impact on your metabolism and muscle biochemistry. This is related to your insulin sensitivity and your blood sugar. If you train on an empty stomach, your glycogen (or stored carbohydrates) is depleted. This means that you are burning more fat.

For best results, eat protein after your workout. This will strengthen and maintain your muscles. It will also promote better recovery. It is advisable to eat near a modern or intense workout. You also need to drink a more water to stay well hydrated. It is important to maintain the electrolyte level. Coconut water can be helpful for this.

You may feel a little dizzy if you exercise while fasting. If you experience it, take a break. It is important to listen to your body. If you are fasting longer, gentle exercises like Pilates, yoga, or walking may be better. They help burn fat without making you uncomfortable.

Intermittent fasting with keto

Some experts say that if you combine intermittent fasting with the keto diet, you will lose more weight.

What is keto?

The keto diet (or ketogenic diet) is a special way of eating where most of the calories come from healthy fats. The remaining calories come from protein. If anything, very few carbohydrates are consumed in this diet.

This low-carb, high-fat diet encourages your body to burn fat, not sugar, for energy. If your body lacks carbohydrates to perform your daily activities, fat is broken down by the liver. It produces ketones and these are then used as fuel for energy. The process is known as ketosis. Hence the name "Keto".

Like intermittent fasting, keto diets have a number of benefits. They can increase weight loss, lower blood sugar, and improve brain function. Many people say that it helps reduce problems like diabetes and obesity.

When you combine a keto diet with an IF, the time you are in ketosis increases. This could make you feel more energetic and less hungry and speed up your weight loss.

If intermittent fasting is to be successful for you, it must work effectively around your lifestyle. You must be sure that you can maintain your diet for the long term. You can only do this if it suits your needs. Remember that intermittent fasting should make your life easier,

If you do intermittent fasting correctly, you will see the result quickly. Not only do you have to lose weight, but you also have to feel more energetic and healthier. You feel more focused and enjoy a multitude of health and wellness benefits. There are many benefits of IF and one of the most important benefit is longer lifespan

Weight Loss Recipes

Tomato Spinach Soup

A simple tomato with spinach soup.

Ingredients:

- One cup of crushed tomatoes
- Three ounces of fresh chopped spinach
- One cup of finely chopped onions
- Half a cup of chopped celery
- Two finely chopped garlic cloves
- Two tablespoon of olive oil
- Quarter of a cup of chopped basil
- One tablespoon of dried thyme
- One tablespoon of dried oregano
- Two cups of low sodium and fat free vegetable broth
- One tablespoon of balsamic vinegar
- Ground black pepper

First heat up the oil in the pot and add in the garlic, celery and onion. Then saute them until they are softened. After that, sprinkle the oregano and thyme over them. Then add crushed tomatoes along with the vegetable broth. Also add in the spinach and basil. Stir until wilted. Then bring it to a boil, reduce the heat and let it simmer for 20 minutes. After that, add in the balsamic vinegar and season with black pepper.

Cauliflower Soup

Ingredients:

- One medium sized potato, cut into one inch pieces
- One medium sized cauliflower, trim it and cut into smaller pieces
- One thinly sliced celery stick
- Two crushed garlic cloves
- One medium size onion, chopped finely
- One tablespoon of dried thyme
- Two table spoon of canola olive oil
- Quarter cup of chopped fresh parsley
- Four cups of fat free and low sodium broth
- Grounded black pepper

First heat up the oil in a pot. Then add the garlic, celery and onions saute and cook until they are softened, which usually take around 5 minutes. Then sprinkle thyme over the vegetables, add the potato and cauliflower followed by the broth. cook on lower flame. Then add in the parsley and stir. Cover the pot and let it simmer for around 30 minutes.

Cucumber And Cantaloupe Salad

Ingredients:
- One cantaloupe, roughly chopped
- Half large cucumber, peeled and roughly chopped
- Three scallions, fine sliced
- Quarter cup of lime juice
- Quarter cup of chopped cilantro leaves
- Salt and pepper

take a small bowl and mix salt, pepper and lime juice. Leave it aside. Then take another bowl and add cilantro, green onions, cucumber and cantaloupe, mix both together.

Tuna Salad

Ingredients:
- Eight cups romaine, chopped
- Two medium tomatoes, diced
- 2 small cans of chunk light tuna, already drained
- Half cup of pimiento- stuffed green olives, sliced
- Quarter cup of lemon juice
- Half teaspoon of garlic and salt
- Three tablespoons of extra virgin olive oil
- Pepper

Mix the oil, garlic, lemon juice, salt and pepper in a bowl. Then add the romaine, olives and tomatoes. Toss to coat them. add tuna and toss again.

Salmon Burger

Ingredients:
- One small can of salmon, flaked and drained
- Half a cup of onion, chopped
- Three quarter cup of bread crumbs
- Two egg whites, slightly beaten
- One tablespoon of butter
- Salt and pepper
- Lemon Cream Sauce
- One teaspoon of grated lemon zest
- One cup of fat-free sour cream
- Two tablespoon of freshly-squeezed lemon juice
- Half a teaspoon of granulated sugar
- Lemon wedges

Take a bowl and put the lemon juice, lemon zest, sugar and sour cream. Mix them until they are properly blended. Then take another bowl, mix the salmon, onion, egg whites, bread crumbs, salt and pepper. shape them into six patties. Heat up the frying pan over medium heat and melt the butter. Then cook the salmon patties until they are brown on both sides, take them out of the pan to plate. Cover with lemon cream and garnish with lemon wedges.

Tuna Steak With Apricot

Ingredients:
- One tune steak, around 150g of weight
- Eight dried apricots
- One medium size tomato
- Half small red onion
- One tablespoon of balsamic vinegar
- One tablespoon of brandy
- Two table spoon of extra virgin olive oil
- Few leaves of lettuce
- Half a teaspoon of dried thyme
- pepper

chop half tomato and dried apricots. Then put them into a blender with vinegar, olive oil, brandy, thyme and. blend the ingredients until fine. Use the mixture to marinate the tuna for 30 minutes. If you plan to marinate for a long time, then keep it in the fridge and take it out 30 minutes before cooking

After the tuna is properly marinated, slice the onions into strips and fry them lightly for 2 minutes. Then chop up the remaining tomato and fry them together with the rest of the apricots. Then place them on the lettuce leaves.

take out the fish with the marinate sauce and fry it in the same pan that you used to cook the tomato and apricot. Cook each side for 3 minutes and it is ready to be served.

Mustard Chicken

Ingredients:
- Two table spoon of mustard
- Four halved chicken breast, boneless and skinless
- Half a cup of non-fat plain yogurt
- Quarter cup of bread crumbs

Preheat the oven to 350 degrees Fahrenheit. Then coat the baking dish with a vegetable spray. Take a small bowl and mix the mustard and yogurt until they are well blended. Then brush the mixture on both sides of the chicken breast. sprinkle bread crumbs on both side of the chicken and pat them lightly. put the chicken on the baking dish, cover it and into the oven. Bake for around 25 minutes. take it out of the oven and serve immediately.

Fry Chicken And Spring Vegetables

Ingredients:

- Two chicken breasts, each about 150 g
- 100 g broccoli
- 100 g baby sweet corn
- Two medium sized carrots
- Bunch of spring onions
- 34 g of ginger
- a tablespoon of olive oil
- Four blocks of egg pasta
- a glass of black bean sauce

boil water and add the pasta. Cook for about 4 minutes until the pasta is ready. cut the chicken breast into inches. Cut the broccoli. peel the ginger and carrots and cut them. Spring onions should be cut diagonally. Take a second pan, cook and blanch the sweet corn and broccoli in water for 2 minutes. And drain well. Take out a saucepan and heat the oil. Add the chicken and stir for about 8 minutes. Place them on a plate. Then heat the pan and add the onions, ginger and carrot. Stir for 2 minutes now add broccoli and sweet corn. Then add the chicken, black bean sauce and pasta. Stir well and this is ready to be served.

Chicken And Tomatoes

Ingredients:
- one can of tomato
- half a cup of sun-dried tomatoes, chopped
- Four boneless, skinless, cut chicken breast
- clove of garlic
- Three teaspoons of marjoram, chopped
- a tablespoon of red wine vinegar
- eight ounces of Orzo
- 2 teaspoons of extra virgin olive oil
- A cup of water
- Half cup of Romano cheese, finely chopped
- a teaspoon of salt
- a packet of frozen artichoke

First, boil the Orzo in a big pot until it becomes tender. It usually takes about 10 minutes. Then drain the Orzo and rinse. take a blender and add a quarter cup of sun-dried tomatoes, can tomatoes, a cup of water, garlic, vinegar, two teaspoons of marjoram and oil. Then mix it until it becomes striking pieces.

Then season both sides of the chicken breast with salt and pepper. Heat the remaining oil in a large saucepan over medium to high heat. Then put the chicken on flame. Cook until golden on the outside and no longer pink on the inside. It takes about 3 to 5 minutes on each side. Then put it on a plate and cover with aluminum foil to keep it warm.

Get a pan, pour the tomato sauce and heat it till it boils. Then pour half a cup into a small bowl. add the cup of sun-dried tomatoes, orzo, artichoke and six tablespoons of cheese. Stir the mixture until it is heated through, which takes around 1 - 2 minutes. Then divide among 4 plates. put sliced chicken on the divided sauce along with two tablespoons of the reserved tomato sauce and sprinkle some marjoram and cheese.

Fried Halibut With Banana And Orange

Ingredients

- A pound of halibut or white meat
- Half a teaspoon of ground coriander
- Two oranges, peeled, segmented, chopped
- Two ripe bananas
- Half teaspoon of orange zest
- Quarter cup of fresh coriander, chopped
- Two tablespoons of lime juice
- a quarter cup of kosher salt

preheat the oven to 450 degrees Fahrenheit. Then get a baking sheet and lightly brush it with cooking spray. Then cut your fish into 4 portions. mix the salt and cilantro in a small bowl before sprinkling them on both sides of the fish. Then put the fish on the baking sheet. Put in the oven and cook it. Depending on the size of the fish, it takes about 10 minutes. While the fish cooks, take a bowl and mix the orange zest, bananas, coriander, chopped oranges, lime juice, salt and coriander. When the fish is ready, place it on the plate and pour the fruit mixture over the fish.

Chicken Stuffed With Gorgonzola And Prunes

Ingredients:

- 1/4 cup whole grain breadcrumbs
- One third of a cup of crumbled Gorgonzola cheese
- Half a cup of chopped plums
- Four boneless skinless chicken breasts, cut
- teaspoon of thyme, chopped
- half a teaspoon of salt
- Half a teaspoon of ground pepper
- chopped shallot
- teaspoon of extra virgin olive oil
- cup of low sodium chicken broth
- half cup of red wine
- Four teaspoons of all-purpose flour

Get a small bowl and mix the breadcrumbs, half teaspoon of thyme, a quarter cup of plums and the gorgonzola. make a horizontal cut just across the thin edge of the chicken, same across the opposite side. Pour about two and a half spoons of the mixture into each chicken breast. Use toothpicks to seal the breast. Season each side of the chicken breast with salt and pepper.

heat a non-stick pan with a tablespoon of oil over medium to high heat. Then boil the chicken until golden, which takes about 4 minutes on each side. Transfer the chicken to a plate. Then add the oil, the shallot and the teaspoon of thyme to the pan and cook. After a minute, add some water and a cup of plums. Reduce the heat to medium and continue cooking, After 2 minutes, Pour the broth into a small bowl with a little flour and whisk until it is smooth. Then pour it into the pan and continue to cook and stir until it has thickened, which takes about two minutes.

Then reduce the heat to low, put the chicken back in the pan with a sauce and turn it over to brush the sauce. Cover the pan and cook the chicken until it is completely cooked. Put it on a plate, take out the toothpick, slice the chicken and garnish with the sauce.

Baby Tiramisu

Ingredients
- Half teaspoon of vanilla extract
- one tablespoons of powdered jaggery
- Half cup of ricotta, fat-free
- Four tablespoons of strong coffee
- eighth teaspoon of ground cinnamon
- Twelve lady's fingers
- Two tablespoons of sweet and sour chocolate chips, melted

Take a bowl and mix the vanilla, ricotta, cinnamon and jaggery, place six ladyfingers on a bread pan, then sprinkle them with two tablespoons of espresso. Then spread the ricotta mixture over the lady's fingers. put another layer of Ladyfingers and sprinkle it with the remaining coffee. sprinkle with melted chocolate. Place the mixture in the refrigerator until the chocolate is firm. It takes about 30 minutes.

Omelet With Spicy Vegetables

Ingredients:

- One tablespoon of golden flax seeds
- Two tablespoons of milk
- Two large eggs
- Half teaspoon of ground turmeric
- teaspoon of dried herb mixes
- Half teaspoon of ground cumin
- A ball of frozen spinach
- Some frozen peas
- 1 medium cup of mushrooms
- Two tablespoons of grated cheese
- Salt and pepper

put the flax seeds in a coffee grinder and let the seeds pulsate until they are ground. Then whisk the egg in a bowl and add the ground flax seeds, milk, herbs, spices, salt and pepper. Continue wiping until mixed well. heat a non-stick pan with a little oil. Pour part of the mixture and wait 30 seconds before whipping the mixture again. Add the frozen spinach. Keep the omelet loose on the edge of the pan. Then put the frozen peas and sliced mushrooms on the same side of the spinach in the omelet. When the omelet is almost done, sprinkle moist cheese over the mushroom and fold the blank side of the omelette over the cheese. Cook for 1 more minute before serving.

Broccoli Soup

Ingredients:
- Half finely chopped onion
- A branch of finely chopped celery
- A medium-sized potato, peeled cut
- Four cups of chopped broccoli with their stems
- Two tablespoons of olive oil
- A cup of low-fat or non-fat milk
- Two cups of low-sodium, low-fat vegetable or chicken broth

pour the oil into the pan and heat it. Then add the celery and onions and sauté for a few minutes until the onions become brown. Then add the broccoli and potato, then the milk and broth. Bring the mixture to a boil. Then reduce the heat, cover the pan and simmer for 20 minutes to make the vegetables tender. Then stop the heating and allow the mixture to cool. Pour them into a blender and mix. Then pour into the pan to warm them before serving.

Tomato, Ginger And Garlic Soup

Ingredients:

- 2 finely chopped garlic cloves
- A medium sized onion, finely chopped
- 5 tomatoes
- a tablespoon of coriander
- chopped ginger

heat two tablespoons of olive oil in a saucepan over medium heat. Then add the garlic and onions and fry them. add the coriander and mix well. Then add the tomatoes and 2 cups of water. Continue mixing until boiling. Then reduce the heat, cover the pan and simmer for about 20 minutes. stir and simmer for another five minutes. Then take the mixture in a blender. Mix the mixture until it becomes smooth

Cabbage soup

Ingredients:

- 2 Large onions
- 2 Green peppers
- 2 tomatoes
- 1 bunch of Celery
- 1 Cabbage
- 3 Carrots
- 1 packet Mushrooms
- 6-8 cups Water
- Chop the vegetables

saute onions in little oil in a pan Add the other vegetables, add water cook for 30 minutes on medium flame

There is one type of diet where a person eats only Cabbage or drinks only Cabbage soup every alternative day, called Cabbage diet.
This soup helps you to lose weight faster.

After Weight Loss

Live a healthy life

Once you've reached your target weight, you want to know how to keep it so you don't lose all that hard work! Finding out in advance will help you reach the point where you have reached your weight loss goal. You don't want to spoil the celebration you want, and of course, you want to continue your newly discovered healthy lifestyle.

How to maintain average weight?

Losing weight will be the easiest part of the whole process. The real challenge is to stay that way after achieving a goal. The sad truth is that there are no short-term fixes.

You have to develop a new lifestyle. You need to focus on better eating habits and daily exercise habits for the rest of your life.

I know it sounds impossible, most of us hate exercising, but after a while you will love it!

We have to change our habits, Small changes in our daily habits over time can cause quantum changes in our body and our health.

Changing habits

The first thing you need to control is the amount of calories you eat each day. This way you know how your weight loss is going.

Scientists have proven that losing fat is just burning more calories than you eat.

Don't skip meals!

Keep in mind that your body's metabolism sees this as a signal that your body is starving and starting to store fat for reserves. Make sure to keep up with your meals as planned. It can also mean that you are eating too late if you miss a meal at a certain time of the day when you are just hungry.

Eat square meals

Adjust your daily calorie intake. Many people wonder if they should immediately increase their daily calorie intake. It is probably advisable to do this, but gradually. Start with just 250 more calories a day. Weigh yourself after a week. You will probably have lost a little more weight. If so, add another 250 calories and weigh yourself a week later. Repeat these steps until you find that your weight stays the same during the week while you weigh. If you've gained weight, take a few 100 calories at a time until your weight is balanced and stays the same from week to week.

split your calories into the right portions of protein, carbohydrates and fats.

Each meal should contain about 30% of the calories from lean protein and 55% of natural complex carbohydrates. The remaining 15% comes from fat.

Eat frequently

Eating five to six small meals a day, as you have probably learned, is a good thing to continue, as it will keep your metabolism going and make you feel satisfied. It is important to continue as well, because you don't want to fall into the trap of increasing your portion size again if it was a problem before. You will eventually get back to first place. At least you will find some of the weight that you have worked so hard to lose.

Avoid junk food

Do not allow junk food to come in. After developing your healthy habits, why should you ruin them by going back to your old habits and eating junk food? You have discovered many delicious flavors to satisfy all your desires with healthy food. Keep fruits and vegetables up to several servings a day, preferably 6-8.

Daily vitamins

Remember to continue taking your daily vitamins. This way you can make sure that you get all the vitamins you need every day and you can also keep your weight healthy.
Continue to eat a variety of foods. This will help you get all the nutrients and vitamins your body needs to keep it working properly. You feel healthy, energized and protect your body by keeping it healthy. You can choose between whole grains, fruits, vegetables and lean protein.

Exercise

Exercise is probably the most important habit of all. Nutrition is only half the battle; The other half is activities!
Don't be lazy now and drop your workout routine. You have learned what type of training is right for you and probably how you can change it from time to time if you have been instructed by a personal trainer.
Changing your routine is a great idea to avoid boredom and guess your body. As long as you always combine your cardiovascular and muscle training, you will stay fit

and feel strong and healthy, while protecting yourself from the illnesses associated with a healthy diet.

As mentioned earlier, cardio will be your best friend when it comes to weight loss. You can do things like:

- Ride a bike
- Go to jog
- stair climbing
- Skiing
- Swimming

These are all great ways to control weight. Always try to exercise for at least 30 minutes daily.

Water

Keep drinking the water! Remember to drink at least eight glasses of water a day for your body to function properly. Water helps digestion, increases your energy and helps rid your body of toxins in a natural way. You also stay hydrated and healthy.

Lifestyle

· Everyone wants to live a long and healthy life. no one wants to expect serious illnesses. While we cannot predict or prevent every situation, there are ways we can protect ourselves to make our lives more complete and healthier.

· Prevention and early detection are the first things to consider. Most people are afraid to see a doctor or even visit the dentist. However, if you have good doctors and stick to these appointments in your life, stay healthy because your doctor can recognize things that you cannot recognize.

· It is also important to know your family history, as your doctor may check your family for symptoms if you have heart disease or cancer and have tests done regularly.

·   Love the people you are with. Make sure you spend time with those around you every day, such as your spouse, children, other family members, friends and colleagues. Take advantage of the time you spend with other people and cultivate healthy friendships. These relationships are necessary for you to feel fulfilled in life.

·   Get eight hours of sleep. Although many people find it difficult to do this because we can be very busy in our lives, it is really very important to live a happy and healthy life.

·   Find something you are good at. We all have times when we have to do something that we really enjoy, and most of them are things that set us apart. It is usually something that makes us feel good inside and can even be soothing and stress relieving.

·   Manage your stress - don't ignore it!
Everyone has stressors and it is important that we manage our stress so that it does not get out of hand and does not consume us, If you are worried and stressed, it can literally make you sick in different ways. Daily walks can help clear your mind and make sure you don't overload your daily agenda or let others plan your day.

·   Find balance in your life.
Do not try to accept too many projects at work or to be consumed by work. Find a balance so you can enjoy everything else around you, like your hobbies, friends and family.

·   Although financial times can be difficult, it is still very important to find time to spend at least with your family, with whom you work so hard to be safe and to take care of yourself.

· The benefits of staying healthy are limitless. It does not only mean that you are satisfied with your look and that you can adapt to this new outfit. Being healthy is linked to your overall physical, mental and social well-being.

Your physical health

If you keep yourself physically healthy, you can help throughout. Not only can it help you participate in daily activities such as walking, moving and bending, but it also allows you to take care of your loved ones in your area who depend on you.

This can be financially beneficial if you avoid preventable diseases which would be very costly.

Your mental health

if you do not have good mental health, your physical health will also be affected. Many people do not realize how important their mental health is to their general well-being. If you get overwhelmed or if this stress governs your life, it can make you sick.

Stress can increase your blood pressure, which increases the risk of heart attack or stroke. You need to manage your stress positively, for example through exercise, meditation, or therapy. Don't deal with stress that can affect your overall health, such as smoking, drinking, or eating unhealthy foods.

Disease prevention

ensuring a healthy diet is essential to your health and to your health in general. The foods you eat can directly affect your health.

Phytochemicals are important for your health and can prevent things like heart disease, certain types of cancer, diabetes, and high blood pressure. They only occur in certain foods such as berries, spinach, olives and kale. Eat a low-fat diet with lots of fruits and vegetables and whole grains to protect your cardiovascular health.

Longer life

Finding a healthy lifestyle can be an important factor in helping you live a long and healthy life. Although you cannot prevent all health problems and some of them are beyond your control, many of the most important of which you can avoid by living a healthy lifestyle.

The main causes of death are chronic diseases such as diabetes, heart disease, stroke and cancer. You can choose your lifestyle by controlling food, keeping your weight at a healthy level, exercising and managing the stressors in your life.

A healthy lifestyle can also improve your mood and give you more self-esteem and mental focus. You will be stronger, have more endurance and will be able to sleep better.

Other benefits of a healthy lifestyle include better digestion and lower blood pressure. Keeping yourself healthy will also help relieve or eliminate back problems and back pain, improve your posture, improve coordination and balance, and lower your resting heart rate.

It is human nature to seek quick solutions. However, when it comes to losing fat, there are no shortcuts.

It's easy to get involved in the hottest diet craze, the latest workout gadget, the hottest class, or the latest pill, but the results they produce are often short-lived at best. If it sounds too good to be true, it probably is.